HEALTH SECRETS FOR THE 21st CENTURY

Volume One

Nutritional Solutions for Health and Longevity

K.W. PETERS

NutriStart Vitamin Company, Victoria, B.C.

E-mail: info@nutristart.com

ISBN:

Printed and bound in Canada
Written by Kenneth Walter Peters
Edited by Vyvyan Rousseaux
Author's Photo by Sarah Brooks
Book Design: BookDesign.ca

Dedicated to Wally Peters

Who started me on the path.

Contents

PART TWO:

SUPPLEMENTS FOR GENERAL HEALTH AND WELL BEING

INTRODUCTION

Like it or not, life is not as simple as it used to be. There was a time when all food was "Health Food" and all produce was organic. Now it's confusing trying to keep up with what's good for you and what is no longer good for you. First butter is a good food, then margarine is better for you than butter; then it is not. Coconut oil is a saturated fat and therefore bad for you, along with all saturated fats. Not so. Now heated polyunsaturated vegetable oils are bad for you, producing trans-fatty acids, and saturated oils are acceptable and even healthful (especially for cooking purposes).

Chocolate is back on the map (as is red wine), but carob, once the preferred health alternative to chocolate, is off the map, because of the bad fats used to bind it together in bar form. The fat in chocolate is now considered to be a safe, naturally saturated fat, and the antioxidant profile of chocolate is high enough to recommend it as a health food, as long as there is more chocolate involved than sugar (minimum 70% cocoa).

Artificial sweeteners are healthier than sugar. Or not. And so on.

These days it is a part-time job to stay ahead of the game and not be confused by marketing hype, misinformation, and disinformation, which is more common than you might assume. When we read often enough about another vitamin or herb that is "proven" to be ineffective or dangerous, eventually we throw up our hands in disgust and go back to our old, bad dietary habits. Over time vitamin A, vitamin C, vitamin E and now calcium supplements, have all had their reputations questioned, and yet these nutrients are all essential to good health. They are all well researched and generally safe: when you know how to use them correctly.

Here is where the "secrets" of the title come in. In essence, I offer balanced and unbiased information that is not commonly known, even among those who use supplements on a regular basis. Certainly those selling you supplements are, unfortunately, not going tell you the advantages of not using their product every day; that is contrary to the purpose of marketing. Indeed, most of the information that modern supplement consumers get is in the form of marketing and free magazines. You get the quality of information that you pay for, in this case. The free magazines have most of their content written by their advertisers, and the publishers seldom critically analyze any claims by the advertisers, for fear of losing advertising dollars.

Knowing how to supplement safely, however, requires reading and research to be done by each individual. We now, more than ever, must take responsibility for our own health, and that means educating ourselves. And, to be effective, this education must be ongoing. Part of the problem appears to be that, even in the area of natural healing, once professionals complete their education they seem to stop keeping up with the latest developments in their fields. I see this with not only doctors (especially in a country with socialized medicine) but also with naturopaths, who are the most important alternative to allopathic doctors. In a vitamin store: forget about it. You will get 3 different answers talking to 3 different salespeople, and different recommendations from different stores.

I am here to tell you how to use supplements correctly. What makes me a better choice for guidance? Knowledge and experience. I have been studying in the natural healing field for almost 30 years and doing nutritional consulting for some 20 years. I have as well experimented on my family and myself for decades, I have been in the field seeing the same people over the years and getting constant feedback from clients, as to what works and what doesn't. Combined with years of lectures and readings, discussions with co-workers trained in other fields (homeopathy, Chinese medicine, energy medicine, herbology, etc), engaging sales representatives in detailed analysis of their products, and my own projects, including writing, research and product design in the field, I have the ideal "generalist" overview, rather than the narrow "specialist" perspective. This allows me to bring you some clarity and common sense to the, sometimes, confusing area of nutritional supplementation.

Overview is the key. Having some knowledge over a broad range of subjects allows one to make links that are often invisible to specialists. It also allows one to mix modalities when attempting to help people to heal themselves. Ailments are often a combination of issues involving body, mind and spirit. Spirit gets overlooked in a secular society, or given too much credence in a religious one, but there is no escaping the fact that if you have no sense of purpose and get no personal satisfaction from your work or from your life, you will have a sense of "dis-ease," which will eventually manifest itself in physical symptoms.

Often, people who use vitamins and supplements excessively are trying to offset this sense of dis-ease, but nothing ever works because the underlying cause is never addressed. Love does not come in a pill, but a caring consultant who hears your story can often be of more value than the pill actually purchased. Such people keep returning to purchase supplements because of the relationship they have with the consultant, which satisfies an essential human need for psycho-nourishment. A need that doctors used to help fill in the old days, before walk-in clinics and ten-minute turnaround visits.

Aside from these emotional needs, there is no denying that our food is lacking nutrients that were once present, and our environment is providing toxins that once were never there. Most physical ailments come down to a lack of specific nutrients and/or an excess of certain toxins. Physical ailments wear down the personality: it is hard to be happy, let alone be pleasant, when you are in pain. Poor personality characteristics lead to isolation, which leads to psychological and spiritual malaise. And, of course psychological and spiritual aberrations will manifest in physical symptoms. It is much easier to heal physical problems than ones that occur in the more subtle realms. The information provided here, for the most part, will only help within the physical realm. It is up to you to fulfill the other needs, which will be easier to do when you feel good.

DISCLAIMER

This book is not intended to diagnose, treat or prescribe. That is the field of specialists (get a second opinion). This book (the first in a series of three) is designed to arm you with some of the most important data for surviving the 21st Century in good health. It is based on a series of newsletters written for NutriStart Vitamin Company, that I design nutritional products for. The material is representative of current beliefs in the natural health fields, processed through the filter of my experience and ongoing research. It is presented in an accessible layman's format, and so will not include footnotes, nor an excessive amount of scientific reference points. Anything you find debatable is easily researched online (see PubMed web address at the end of chapter one), where you will find arguments both for and against any specific subject. Ultimately, we all look at both sides of the research and make up our own minds. Keep open to changing your mind, if and when new evidence or ideas present themselves. And they will.

PART ONE:

THE BASICS OF SUPPLEMENTATION

Many of you may, of course, already use the following "basic" supplements, yet you may not be aware of certain issues that accompany them. For example, the problem with taking too many B-vitamins, the mistaken information on the dangers of too much vitamin A, the preferred form of vitamin C, or the latest advances in the recommended use of vitamin E. Not to mention, the recently discovered dangers of ingesting too much calcium and not enough magnesium. So, in this section, we will take an in-depth look at vitamins A, B, C, D, E, F (Fatty Acids), and the main minerals.

Most of us begin our journey into the vitamin realm with the purchase of a one-a-day-multiple vitamin and mineral mix. While this is a good beginning it does come up short, since no one tablet can provide sufficient quantities of all the supplements required, especially vitamin C, vitamin E, calcium and magnesium. Were these nutrients to be included at adequate levels in one pill, it would be impossible to swallow.

GENDER DIFFERENCES

Let's begin our hypothetical journey by assuming that you search for the best one-a-day "multiple" that you can find, perhaps narrowing down the choices to one that is gender specific. Such a formulation will provide extra iron for women and extra zinc for men, as this is the only essential difference in basic nutritional requirements between genders. This is because women lose iron during menstruation and men lose zinc during ejaculation.

Gender and age specific formulas aimed at men and post-menopausal women generally do not include iron, since excess iron has been linked to heart disease. This is because too much iron in the tissues leads to free radical production and depletes the body of the antioxidant vitamin E. If you eat red meat and you are a male, or a female past menstruation, it is a good idea to avoid iron as a supplement, unless you have been diagnosed as iron-deficient. Some iron is however included in multi-vitamins that are aimed at "active" men, as it is assumed that they will sweat out iron (along with other minerals, most obviously the "electrolytes") due to vigorous exercise.

This fear of iron is in fact based on an old Finnish study, where all the people in the study were big meat eaters (2 or 3 times daily), and those with the highest iron levels had the most heart disease. Unless you are yourself a big meat eater, worries about iron intake may be unnecessary. (Remember that, aside from fatigue, the other main symptom of iron deficiency is often feeling cold, especially when the others around you do not feel cold.)

CHAPTER ONE

VITAMIN A, SUNGLASSES AND ASTHMA

I have found vitamin A deficiency to be one of the top three or four most common nutritional deficiencies that I see on a regular basis, while doing nutritional consulting.

A high quality "one-a-day" can provide enough vitamin A for basic needs if, and this is a big if, it uses natural beta-carotene. Unfortunately 90% of the time the beta-carotene provided is in a synthetic form, which renders it essentially worthless. Natural beta-carotene, a viable supplement, will be listed on the label as "natural" or will include a list of the "mixed carotenoids" that accompany it in a natural complex. If the label simply states "Beta carotene" then it is synthetic.

My first clue to a person's need for extra vitamin A is to ascertain if they need to use sunglasses. A little known sign of vitamin A deficiency is squinting in the sun. When I am consulting with clients who have lung or sinus problems, I will suggest that they take extra vitamin A until they no longer squint on a sunny day. Inevitably, they usually say that they always squint, or they thought that everyone squints on a bright day. My response is that no tropical culture found it necessary to invent sunglasses until modern times, now they are prevalent, as is the rise of asthma.

IMPORTANCE OF VITAMIN A

The link between sunglasses and asthma is that of vitamin A deficiency, which leads to an erosion of the internal mucosal membranes. From the eyes (helping with dry eye, night vision, color sensitivity) to the anus, vitamin A builds and maintains mucosal membranes. This includes the lining of your sinuses, throat, lungs, intestines and more. This lining is your first line of defense against potentially invasive allergens, bacteria and pollutants from the outside world.

If these particles get through that defensive line, symptoms such as chronic sinus problems, allergies, interstitial cystitis, asthma and other lung and bronchial ailments will occur. Food allergies happen, in part, when the lining of the gut has been further compromised by Candida yeast overgrowth (linked to antibiotic overuse and birth control pills), or by Crohn's disease and colitis. In fact, one study showed that women with vaginal candidiasis ("yeast infection") had extremely low beta-carotene levels in their blood (one sixth of the average.) (Mikhail MS, et al., Decreased beta-carotene levels in exfoliated vaginal epithelial cells in women with vaginal candidiasis. Am J Reproductive Immunol 32, 221-225, 1994) This makes sense, from the point of view that sufficient beta-carotene would necessary to make enough vitamin A to thicken and protect the vaginal lining.

Now here is where it gets dicey; I will commonly recommend 30,000IU (fat-soluble nutrients are generally measured in "IU" or "international units") of vitamin A daily. This natural form is usually derived from fish liver oil, mainly from halibut, as it is about four times higher in vitamin A, than cod liver oil. (When purchasing such a product, ensure that it is from a reliable vitamin company, and that the product has been processed in such a manner as to eliminate any toxins from the fish liver.) For strict vegetarians, vitamin A also seems to be somewhat effective in its synthetic form ("retinyl palmitate"), unlike beta-carotene, which, as we will see, is useless in synthetic form.

These pills come in strengths of 10,000IU, so one takes 3 pills daily, with a meal containing some fat. If the client is not already taking a vitamin D supplement (now commonly recommended as an anti-cancer agent), I will suggest that they choose a "Mega Halibut Oil" pill, which includes 400IU of vitamin D with the 10,000IU of vitamin A. This is because vitamin D also plays a role in maintenance of the mucosal membranes. (More on this later.)

IS IT DANGEROUS?

The dicey part is that most people have been made afraid of vitamin A by distorted media attention. Women are told not to get more than 5,000IU daily, in case they get pregnant and increase their risk of birth defects, and seniors are warned that more than 3,000IU daily can contribute to osteoporosis.

I disagree. I've followed up on these studies (links to follow) and in fact more birth defects are caused worldwide by vitamin A deficiency, than excess. Of course vitamin A deficiency is extremely common in the developing world, but it also turns out to be fairly common in the West as well. We'll get to why that is in a moment.

Let's have a closer look at the original study linking high doses of vitamin A to birth defects, published in October 1995 in the New England Journal of Medicine. In the developing fetus vitamin A is necessary for regulating organ development and for normal cellular differentiation. Those women who were taking more than 10,000IU of vitamin A daily during the first trimester were 2.4 time more likely to have children with birth defects ("cranio-facial deformities"), and those ingesting more than 20,000IU were four times more likely to have babies with birth defects.

While this sounds appalling from one perspective, there is another way to look at these figures. When observing the 57 women consuming large doses of vitamin A we see that only one baby in

57 developed defects, whereas 56 did not. So one wonders if we can even blame the vitamin A for this anomaly. The experts did go on to state elsewhere that "We know of no reason for anyone to avoid eating carrots, tomatoes, or other carotene-containing foods, and we know of no adverse effect associated with beta-carotene dietary supplements."

With regards to the idea that vitamin A contributes to osteoporosis, that study is countered by another (see below), and the fact that vitamin A is necessary for bone growth.

A DEFICIENCY IN THE WEST

Why would we, one of the best-fed peoples in the world, be deficient in vitamin A? Well, because our main source of dietary vitamin A was consuming cow's liver. When is the last time you had a tasty serving of liver and fried onions? When I was a kid we had liver once or twice weekly, giving us on average 30,000 to 60,000IU of vitamin A weekly. The livers (and other organs) of mammals, fowl and fish used to be consumed on a regular basis by humans everywhere, providing adequate vitamin A levels. The French still consume goose liver pate (94 grams of goose liver contains 29,138IU of vitamin A), which may be part of the famous "French Paradox."

For those unfamiliar, the "French Paradox" is based on the observation that, while the French consume more saturated fat that Americans, they have less heart disease. This has been attributed to their intake of red wine and the antioxidants it provides, and possibly to the fact that their saturated fat comes from natural sources, such as meat and dairy, whereas the American diet provides fat mostly in the form of damaged vegetable oils (more on this in Chapter 7). Currently, our main source of A would be as beta-carotene in a fresh glass of carrot juice, or in yellow and orange fruits and vegetables.

My usual suggestion is that people take 30,000IU daily for a few weeks, or until they stop squinting in the sun. They then should roll back to 10,000IU daily, while skipping weekends, raising the dose if they find themselves squinting again. This recommendation fully acknowledges that I am not a naturopath but simply a nutritional consultant. I met a young woman, however, whose naturopath told her to take 100,000IU per day for a month, so my recommendations are conservative compared to some.

Doses from 50,000IU to 100,000IU, for a few months, are often used to treat stubborn acne (there is a synthetic acne drug which amounts to much the same thing, but has dangerous side effects). Many texts indicate that toxicity of vitamin A occurs at 50,000IU daily for a year. I have even seen a study done with infants being treated for respiratory viral ailments, where they were given 25,000IU of vitamin A daily, for a short period. In this case the infants were, in fact, given "micellized" vitamin A, which is a water-soluble form (available mostly in pharmacies).

Now these suggestions are for people in general good health. Those with liver damage, renal failure, and alcoholics, should not use high doses without the advice of a professional. Women who are pregnant should obviously also err on the side of caution and avoid more than 5,000IU of fat-soluble vitamin A. When we use a water-soluble form of vitamin A, however, such as micellized, there are no worries, since the body can easily excrete what it does not use, unlike the fat-soluble fish liver oils, which are stored in the body, mostly in the liver.

BETA CAROTENE

This water-soluble tenancy is also true of beta-carotene, which is known as "pro-vitamin A." What this means is that the body will convert beta-carotene into vitamin A until it has enough vitamin A, and the extra will then serve as an anti-oxidant, fighting off the damaging effects of free radicals. But, beta-carotene requires adequate zinc in order to convert to vitamin A in the body, and those with diabetes and hypothyroid conditions lack the ability to convert beta-carotene into vitamin A in their bodies. These people, and those who take very large amounts of beta-carotene, may find their skin turning a mild shade of orange. Even those who drink copious amounts of carrot juice will observe this effect and, in fact, some natural tanning pills are made up mostly of high levels of carotenoids.

The problem with beta-carotene is that most of the products on the market are worthless, or worse. You may have heard that smokers are advised to not take beta-carotene, as it could increase their cancer risk. In fact, vitamin A can help prevent cancer in smokers by healing lung damage and rebuilding the little hairs (cilia) lining the lungs that clean them of particles. This warning about beta-carotene and smokers is based on a Finnish study done a few decades ago. In this study (involving a lot of smokers) those on the high beta- carotene regimen were found to have marginally more (18%) cancer than those on the placebo. ("The Alpha-tocopherol, Beta –carotene Cancer Prevention Study Group, The effect of vitamin E and beta-carotene on incidence of lung cancer and other cancers in male smokers." N Engl J Med 330, 1029-1035, 1994.)

The seldom-mentioned reason for this outcome was the fact that the study used only synthetic beta-carotene. Original studies showing benefits of beta-carotene were based on checking the blood levels of beta-carotene in people who obtained it from food. Population studies consistently show a strong protective effect from dietary carotene intake against a wide variety of cancers, including cervix, gastrointestinal, lung, skin and uterus. (Ziegler RG, "A review of the epidemiologic evidence that carotenoids reduce the risk of cancer." J Nutr 119, 116-122, 1989.)

Natural beta-carotene exists with a family of other carotenoids, including alpha carotene, which is ten times more powerful as an antioxidant than the beta form, along with other co-factors such as lutein and zeaxanthin. Because beta-carotene is very prone to oxidative damage researchers have observed that other antioxidant nutrients need to be present with it, for it to be effective. Thus we find in this Finnish study that the group that received both beta-carotene and vitamin E did not show any increase in cancer levels. This is a perfect example of why some studies done on antioxidants show negative effects (which are then widely disseminated in the press). As we will discuss later, antioxidants need to be considered a "family" of nutrients and to be taken in conjunction with one another.

A good product containing natural beta-carotene, will list the other carotenoids on the label as well (a reasonable dose of a natural beta-carotene product is 25,000IU daily). Unfortunately, most multi-vitamins still use the synthetic form because it is a cheaper raw material, meaning that, along with their low levels of actual vitamin A (2,500IU to 5,000IU), a multivitamin will seldom provide the minimum requirement of vitamin A.

OTHER FUNCTIONS OF VITAMIN A

Like most nutrients, vitamin A has a host of functions. Protein requires vitamin A in order to be utilized by the body. Vitamin A prevents night blindness and other eye problems. Deficiencies of vitamin A can also manifest as dry hair or skin, dry eyes, reproductive difficulties, sinusitis or pneumonia. Vitamin A is a powerful immune stimulant, especially protective against respiratory infections because the mucosal membranes (comprised of epithelial cells) function as a physical barrier against infections. Vitamin A also stimulates both T-cells and the antibody-producing B-cells, so well, that one study showed that high doses of vitamin A improved the health of infants with HIV infections.

WARNINGS

Substances that interfere with vitamin A absorption include antibiotics, laxatives and some cholesterol-lowering drugs.

Vitamin A overdose symptoms include, ironically, dryness of

the mucous membranes, as well as hair loss, chronic headaches, vomiting, and liver damage. Yet, I have to wonder if we are misinformed on the warnings to people with liver damage. Consider that the liver stores 90% of vitamin A, yet the majority of us are deficient in this nutrient. Since it is anti-viral and fights infection, perhaps those with Hepatitis or Cirrhosis of the liver would actually have been protected by vitamin A, if their livers were full of it.

Recent studies have indicated that vitamin A at high levels may deplete vitamin D from the body. Since these two vitamins co-exist in the livers of animals, this interdependency is logical, and I would suggest that the safest approach is to include 1000IU of vitamin D for every 10,000IU of vitamin A. (This does not apply to beta-carotene.) This relationship does not appear to occur in the reverse, indicating that high levels of vitamin D do not require high levels of vitamin A. Yet again, logic would indicate that if we are going to take high levels of vitamin D, we should probably ensure that we are getting at least a modicum of vitamin A.

TOPICAL USE

One interesting piece of anecdotal information came from a client of mine who was in her fifties, but had the facial appearance of being in her thirties. She told me that for the last fifteen years she had been opening a capsule of vitamin A (10,000IU) every night and applying it to her face. I have tried this and the skin does indeed absorb the vitamin A, as opposed to vitamin E, which lays rather heavily upon the skin, when used in such a fashion. Vitamin A is noticeably healing to the skin and useful for nebulous skin conditions that are undefined but troublesome. When I apply vitamin A to my skin I usually dilute it in a small amount of Jojoba or Rosehip Seed oil, both of which are also helpful for aging skin.

Below are some links for those wishing to do a little more research. As mentioned earlier, in the natural health field, as with conventional medicine, one must take responsibility for one's own health; build your knowledge and get to know your own body. Only by being actively involved in our health and well-being will we be able to maintain it.

FOLLOWING THE SCIENCE

To find the studies I have used, in part, to confirm this alternative thesis that vitamin A deficiency is widespread in the Western world, and not dangerous to take in moderately high amounts, enter the following study titles into the PubMed (an archive of medical studies from around the world) search engine (www.pubmed.gov). Following each title I will summarize their conclusions.

1. "Serum retinoids and beta-carotene as predictors of hip and other fractures in elderly women." CONCLUSION: We found no evidence to support any skeletal harm associated with increased serum indices of retinal exposure or modest retinal supplementation in this population.
2. "Vitamin A and beta-carotene supply of women with gemini or short birth intervals: a pilot study." CONCLUSION: Despite the fact that vitamin A and beta-carotene rich food is generally available, risk groups for low vitamin A supply exist in the Western world.
3. "Vitamin A deficiency disorders in children and women." CONCLUSION: While reductions of child mortality (in the developing world) of 19-54% following vitamin A treatment have been widely reported, more recent work suggests that dosing newborns with vitamin A may, in some settings, lower infant mortality. Among women, one large trial has so far reported a (roughly) 40% reduction in mortality related to pregnancy with weekly, low-dose vitamin A supplementation."

CHAPTER TWO

THE SUNSHINE VITAMIN THAT YOU'RE PROBABLY NOT GETTING FROM THE SUN

"I think vitamin D is introducing a golden age of medicine."

Cedric Garland, professor of preventive medicine, University of California.

Also critical to maintaining our internal lining of the body and its organs is vitamin D. No "one-a-day" is going to provide sufficient vitamin D, as Health Canada only allows a maximum of 1,000IU in a daily multivitamin, and most brands still only provide the old standard amount of 400IU. But, scientists now believe that a host of ailments, as well as perhaps up to 80% of all cancers (those which occur on the lining of organs,) are due to a chronic deficiency in vitamin D. Some of those scientists currently ingest 8,000IU of D daily, while others prescribe up to 10,000IU for treating depression in the winter. While this may sound insanely high, the fact is that you can produce 10,000IU of vitamin D within one half hour of sunbathing.

Known today as the "sunshine vitamin", in past decades vitamin D was known as the "anti-rachitic vitamin" due to its use as a treatment for rickets (a disease causing bones to become soft and bendable, leading to bowed legs, knock knees and other bone malformations). These days the "winter blahs" and the longing for a sunny tropical vacation may be more modern indicators of a vitamin D deficiency. It's been estimated that as many as 80% of Canadians may have dangerously low levels of vitamin D, during our long winters. The supplement is now being prescribed for such problems as low energy, depression and joint pain. And it seems that almost daily a new link between vitamin D deficiency and another ailment is found, even celiac disease (gluten-sensitivity) appears to be indirectly linked to a deficiency of vitamin D.

WHAT DOES "D" DO?

Vitamin D is a fat-soluble nutrient that functions as both a vitamin and a hormone. Active metabolites of vitamin D are produced in the liver and kidney, and affect other tissues, primarily the intestinal mucosa and bone tissue. Until recently, it was believed that the only important function of vitamin D was to increase absorption of calcium and to increase calcium deposition into the bones. Then, it was found that cultures below the equator had very little incident of Multiple Sclerosis, yet when those same peoples moved north of the equator, their levels rose to the same as those residing in the northern countries. (Extreme northern dwellers, such as the Inuit, obtained their vitamin D primarily from eating fish and mammal livers.)

A recent issue of the Journal of the American Medical Association published a study done on Caucasian members of the U.S. Military. In this study the soldiers with the highest levels of vitamin D were 62% less likely to develop M.S. than those with low levels. (No link was found between African Americans or Hispanics, possibly since there were so few in the study and possibly because dark skin doesn't absorb sunlight as readily as pale skin.) Dr. William Finn, a vitamin D expert at the University of North Carolina stated "There is no question that vitamin D deficiency is an epidemic in the U.S." and this study was "just one more reason to pay attention to it."

VITAMIN D AND CANCER

Before long a link between low vitamin D levels and prostate cancer was established. "Our findings suggest that vitamin D plays an important protective role against prostate cancer, especially ... aggressive disease," said Haojie Li, MD, PhD, a researcher at Brigham and Women's Hospital and Harvard University School of Public Health, in a recent news release. Researchers found that men with the highest levels of vitamin D had significantly lower overall risk (45%) of devolping prostate cancer. Currently a study is under way to test a high dose vitamin D product (DN-101: Calcitriol) in conjunction with a chemotherapy drug, for treating those with prostate cancer. Clinicians hope to increase survival times and improve quality of life in those cancer patients studied, and have already noted that the patients have at least found the chemotherapy easier to tolerate.

Another new study, published by the American Journal of Preventive Medicine, explored the link between blood levels of vitamin D and the risk of colon cancer, observing 1500 individuals over 25 years. They found that a daily intake of 2,000IU of vitamin D3 could reduce the incidences of colorectal cancers by two-thirds. It has already been observed for some time now that death rates from breast, colon, ovarian and prostate cancer, are considerably lower in countries with sunnier climates. Certainly, people diagnosed with cancer during the summer show a better prognosis than persons who are diagnosed during the winter.

Now, a new breast cancer study has found that individuals with the highest blood levels of vitamin D had the lowest risk of breast cancer. (Journal of Steroid Biochemistry and Molecular Biology) Dr. Cedric Garland of the University of California, San Diego, went so far as to state: "It has more potential than any other vitamin or micronutrient to prevent cancer." The doctors went on to say that by taking 2,000IU of vitamin D3 daily, one could maintain a serum blood level of "D" associated with a 50% reduction in breast cancer risk. They then suggest that spending 10 to 15 minutes daily in the sun will accomplish this. (I will cover sunbathing further on.)

WHY IS "D" SO IMPORTANT?

Professor Garland believes that the root of the cancer epidemic in the Western world is due to insufficient levels of vitamin D. This is based in part on the theory of evolution. Since our species evolved near the equator, we still have many of our biological processes calibrated to that level of vitamin D. Having migrated northward, where the sunlight is weak during the fall and winter, we've upset our vitamin D metabolism leading to ailments now linked to insufficient vitamin D levels. The fact that diseases that are seemingly unrelated, like cancer, diabetes and multiple sclerosis, can all be caused by vitamin D deficiency, underscores the theory that the vitamin works like a master switch, turning genes on and off. In fact hundreds of different genes may be regulated by vitamin D since, according to John White from McGill University in Montreal, "virtually every cell in the body has receptors for vitamin D".

Especially interesting to me, is the fact that one of the key functions of vitamin D is to maintain healthy epithelium, those cells which line the outside of our organs, and the inside of our body. Though these tissues lining the body are only a fraction of the weight of the body, they account for about 85% of all cancers, known as carcinomas. This includes breast, colon, pancreas, prostate and uterus cancer. The other forms of cancer, known as sarcomas, strike in muscles and connective tissue, and don't have an association with vitamin D deficiency. Each organ has cells that depend on the vitamin D to sustain them, so for example, if the lung lining can no longer repulse bacteria it may be susceptible to tuberculosis. A weakening of the glial cells in the nervous system could manifest as multiple sclerosis, and a weakening of the islet cells on the pancreas can lead to diabetes.

VITAMIN A WORKS WITH "D"

Those who have followed my work know that I consider vitamin A to be one of the most common nutritional deficiencies in the West. And one of the main functions of vitamin A is the building of the lining of all the internal mucosal membranes. So we know, that both these nutrients keep our insides healthy and protected from the outside world, and we know that nature provides them together, where they are found in the livers of mammals and fish. I believe, that the combination of restorative levels of vitamins A and D together, may indeed usher in a "golden age of medicine".

One of the main functions of epithelial cells in this lining is to forbid the entrance of bacteria and viruses that cause infection in the body. As our vitamins A and D decline and the barrier thins, tissues are exposed to attack from agents of disease. It has already been established that vitamin D will help fight infectious diseases of the lungs, such as influenza and tuberculosis. It is only recently, that a scientist came up with the convincing thesis that influenza rates rise in the winter because our levels of vitamin D fall.

SUNBATHING

For years, we have been advised to stay out of the sun excessively to avoid getting skin cancer. Ironically, it now appears, that a deficiency of vitamin D may also be linked to skin cancer, as well as the aforementioned forms of cancer. The Cancer Society currently suggests that you get "some" sun, but not "too much." Researchers now maintain that even though there may be some risk of skin cancer from over exposure to sunlight, the benefits of preventing the difficult, hard to treat cancers, outweighs the risk of getting the relatively easier to treat skin cancer.

Regarding skin cancer, we should consider the option of the

tanning booth. While most authorities advise against it due to the increased risk of skin cancer, it is an ideal way to strongly boost natural vitamin D levels. One first should make sure that the tanning salon uses "medium-pressure" lamps, which put out UVB rays. Some tanning booths only use "high-pressure" lamps, which put out only UVA rays and will not produce vitamin D in the skin. One expert suggests that the safe way to use such a tanning bed is to only stay for half the time recommended for tanning, and to wear a sunscreen on your face during the process. The face is the part of the body least effective at producing vitamin D, something worth remembering, if that is the only part of your body exposed to the sun during your outdoor activities.

It was previously assumed that we got plenty of vitamin D from our limited exposure to natural sunlight, and so the medical profession still maintains that 10 to 15 minutes is sufficient. We now know that this is not necessarily so; that is, unless you run around naked and dirty, most of the time.

WHY YOU MIGHT NOT BE GETTING VITAMIN D FROM THE SUN

Making vitamin D from the sun is not as simple as we originally thought. The process begins when oils, produced by your skin, are irradiated by ultraviolet rays from the sun. An inactive sterol, formed from cholesterol, then converts to the substance "cholecalciferol." At this point, the compound enters the blood, through the skin, where it is both converted into an active form of vitamin D, and stored in the liver. Later, the kidneys will get involved releasing an enzyme, which turns the somewhat active D into its most potent form. The kidneys decide how much vitamin D to convert into this most biologically active form (for immediate utilization by the body), based on the levels of sodium and potassium in the blood.

When we eat local foods, the levels of sodium and potassium they contain varies from summer to winter. Even among the Inuit in the far north, potassium intake will be higher in the warmer months, and sodium levels higher in the darker months. This fact supports the oriental concept of eating what grows where you live, when it is in season. When we eat a banana (very high in potassium) we essentially tell the kidneys that it is high summer (or that we are in the tropics), and thus it has no need to rally vitamin D, because we must be getting a lot of sun. Clearly, our modern eating practices would have worsened our already widespread deficiency in vitamin D. In addition, anyone with liver or kidney disorders can have a further impairment of vitamin D production in their body.

Other modern conventions also have reduced our vitamin D intake. For example, creating vitamin D in the skin from sunlight is restricted by skin pigments, so dark-skinned people immigrating to northern countries, would be at a disadvantage. As well, synthetic sun block products screen out ultraviolet light. Sun block with an SPF of only 8 will inhibit more than 95% of vitamin D production in the skin. Clothing, smoke, fog, smog, and most glass, screen out the UV light and interfere with vitamin D formation.

EXCESS BATHING

Then there is the daily shower. Consider how unnatural the daily hot bath is for the human animal (with a few exceptions, including the Romans and the Japanese at certain points in their history). For most of history, the majority of humans could only bath occasionally (if they didn't fear it as unhealthy), ensuring that aside from lice and fleas, we at least had good amounts of vitamin D. By the time a bather emerges from that hot, chlorine and detergent mix, all the oils on the surface of the skin have been washed away. Moisturizer does not serve the same function, as far as the creation of vitamin D is concerned, as the oils that we naturally produce are cholesterol-based.

Not only that, but we also damage the protective acid mantle of friendly bacteria which resides on our skin. This can contribute to unhealthy skin conditions. And then there is the additional problem of inhaling chlorine gas everyday, especially since chlorine is what is known as a "cumulative carcinogen." That means that, like radiation, it is not how much you get in a sitting, but how much you store over decades. One shower is evidently equal to drinking a days' worth of chlorinated water, since chlorine absorbs more readily through the lungs than the stomach. (This can be avoided by purchasing a carbon-based shower filter, commonly available at hardware and some drug stores.)

Still, it is suggested that a Caucasian could generate enough vitamin D, by exposing 50% of the (unwashed) skin to 15minutes of noontime sun on a clear day. Those with darker pigment would require at least twice as long under the same conditions, since the melanin in their skin acts as a sunscreen. At Canadian latitudes, during the fall and winter, sunlight is too weak to cause any vitamin D production. Usually, if your shadow is longer than you are, it means that there is not enough sunlight to produce vitamin D in your body.

SUPPLEMENTING WITH VITAMIN D

Supplemental vitamin D is usually defined as ergocalciferol (D2, made from ultraviolet irradiated yeast) and cholecalciferol (D3, derived from ultraviolet irradiation of lanolin from sheep's wool, or from fish liver oil). It is now believed that only the D3 form is active, and so should be your choice when purchasing a supplemental form. As far as dietary sources of vitamin D, the common dietary source is believed to be vitamin D-fortified milk (other dairy products are not fortified), which provides only about 100IU of vitamin D per cup. Most people do not realize that when low-fat dairy products are consumed, the vitamin D is mostly removed, since it resides in the fat component.

Vitamin D is found naturally occurring in the livers of most creatures (though seldom eaten anymore), in the edible portion of oily fish (including salmon, herring and sardines), egg yolk and butter. A 4 oz serving of wild salmon (sockeye) can provide over 700IU of vitamin D, but pacific salmon and farmed salmon offer only half the amount of vitamin D. A serving of sardines contains nearly 600IU, while an egg yolk provides only about 25IU of D. Since plants are a poor source of vitamin D, strict vegetarians who cannot get daily exposure to sunlight require a supplemental form. Up until recently, most people were advised to obtain at least the Recommended Daily Allowance of 400IU of vitamin D from all sources. At the time, it was assumed that sufficient vitamin D could be obtained from sunshine and dairy products.

HOW MUCH TO TAKE

The medical system currently maintains that taking more than 2,000IU of vitamin D per day can cause the body to absorb excessive calcium, possibly damaging the kidneys and liver. In those people prone to kidney stones, high vitamin D levels can elevate their risk, due to increasing the levels of oxalates in their urine. On the other hand, those people naturally treating conditions of Multiple Sclerosis take around 6,000IU of vitamin D per day. (Other important factors for treating MS naturally, include high levels of the methylcobalamin form of sublingual vitamin B-12, up to 60mg daily, high levels of the omega 3 fatty acids from fish, and the removal of mercury fillings from the teeth.)

I am also aware of a physician, Dr. Abram Hoffer (a pioneer in the field of nutrition and recently deceased), who was advising some of his patients with depression to take 10,000IU of vitamin D per day throughout the winter, suggesting that it is the equivalent of a tropical holiday. Studies have been done where seniors have been injected with 50,000IU of vitamin D at the beginning of the winter, and just left to ride it out through the season. Reinhold Bieth from the University of Toronto is Canada's leading vitamin D researcher. Dr. Bieth had been taking 8,000IU of vitamin D daily for years. Even the Canadian Cancer Society has recommended that adults take 1000IU of vitamin D daily in fall and winter (all year round for non-whites). And the Canadian Pediatric Society now calls for pregnant and breastfeeding women to take 2000IU daily in order to prevent childhood diseases. The society also suggests that infants can be given 1,000IU and children 2,000IU, daily.

Personally I take, and recommend, 5000IU of vitamin D daily, going as high as 10,000IU for a few days, depending on the time of year (and my mood in the winter), in a sublingual (under the tongue) form. This recommendation, as with vitamin A, is for only five days a week. We will touch on this approach in more detail later on, but for now, think of it as giving the body a chance to use up any excess of a fat-soluble nutrient that we might have built up.

A gentleman called me concerned that the amount of vitamin D that had been recommended, to him by another consultant, was dangerous. His advisor believes that we need to fill up our deficiency before settling into a moderate daily dose, and so advised this gentleman to take 15,000IU twice daily for 3 to 5 days, before dropping back to 10,000IU for daily use (outside of sunbathing). I assured the man that my research indicated that high doses were quite safe for a week or so, and then inquired as to how he felt. He told me that, after a few days, he had so much energy and such a positive mental attitude, that he felt like a young man again.

VITAMIN D AND THE SKIN

Placing the amounts of vitamin D recommended into perspective, let us consider what nature provides. Humans, deficient in vitamin D, can make at least 10,000IUof vitamin D within 30 minutes of full body exposure to the sun (assuming that you have oils on your skin). The maximum dose of vitamin D is obtained before the skin turns pink. (As a related aside, nude sunbathing will increase testosterone levels in men if their testes are exposed to the sun. Remember that vitamin D is also a hormone, like testosterone.) Historically, even those of us in the northern hemisphere, would have spent considerably more time outdoors than 30 minutes per day.

Now, not all of this 10,000IU of vitamin D would be produced as active D3. Most of it would be stored in the skin as inactive D2, and later it would be drawn upon as needed and converted into the active form, so that the body can utilize it.

Just recently researchers at the University of California, San Diego, found that the skin stores a considerable amount of inactive vitamin D until it is attacked by microbes or bacteria, through a cut, scrape, bite or abrasion. The body then activates the vitamin D, in the skin, converting it into the D3 form in order to defend the skin against these invaders. "Our study shows that skin wounds need vitamin D3 to protect against infection and begin the normal repair process" said Dr. Richard Gallo, in the Journal of Clinical Investigation.

IS IT SAFE?

Toxicity in adults occur when they take 100,000IU daily for a few months. Yet, in the only documented case of pharmacological overdose (www.vitamindcouncil.org), a man inadvertently took between 156,000IU and 2,000,000IU daily for 2 years. Once properly diagnosed, he recovered uneventfully after treatment with steroids and sunscreen. Demineralization of bone mass may occur when the daily dose exceeds 40,000IU daily for a long period of time.

If you suspect you are possibly deficient in vitamin D ask your doctor do a blood test to confirm it. If you choose to take high levels of vitamin D (over 5,000IU) it is a good idea to have a blood test a month later to ensure that you are not mobilizing too much calcium into the bloodstream ("hypercalcemia"). Remember, vitamin D is a fat-soluble vitamin. This means that like other fat-soluble nutrients in pill form (vitamins A, E, K, etc), it is best taken with a meal that contains some fat, for optimal absorption. Because it is fat-soluble, you may take all the pills at one meal. In pill form, the softgel capsule (where the D is in a base of fat) is far more effective than tablets, that don't appear to work well at all. In fact, some authorities believe that it is best absorbed when taken sublingually (dissolved under the tongue).

Almost all the articles I researched end with a warning not to self-prescribe the vitamin, as indicated by the following quote from Dr. Kim Chi (working on the new vitamin D related drug for treating prostate cancer): "We don't want people heading out there and taking boatloads of vitamin D. It can be very toxic and life-threateningly toxic." I disagree.

I suggest, that compared to many of the pharmaceutical drugs casually dumped into the market place, and readily prescribed (until the dangers manifest themselves in us, the real guinea pigs), you could hardly come close to that danger in self-prescribing most nutrients. Do a little research and find out how many people have died from vitamin overdoses in the last decade (only from Iron, in the past, before child-proof lids). Now compare that to the deaths from prescription drugs: 106,000 annually in the U.S. ("a conservative number.") You do the arithmetic and then make your decision.

OTHER POTENTIAL USES FOR VITAMIN D:

ACNE: An old study from 1938 showed a dramatic improvement in patients with severe acne when they were treated with between 5,000IU and 14,000IU of vitamin D daily. (Vitamin A at dosage levels of 50,000IU daily, for a short period, has also been shown to improve severe acne, as has zinc at 50mg per day.)

ASTHMA: Childhood asthma has been linked to maternal vitamin D deficiency by two Harvard studies, and more than one parent has claimed a reversal in symptoms by supplementing their children with vitamin D. I have seen cases of adult asthma symptoms eliminated by moderately high levels of combined vitamin A and D.

AUTISM: U.S. researchers studied the autism rates for children born in California, Oregon and Washington state, from 1987 to 1999, and compared them to the daily precipitation reports. Published in 2008 in the Archives of Pediatrics and Adolescent Medicine, the study concluded: "Autism prevalence rates for school-aged children in California, Oregon and Washington in 2005 were positively related to the amount of precipitation these counties received from 1987 through 2001." In other words, children who lived in the wettest counties were more likely to have autism. Researchers were unclear why this connection occurred, but I would put forth that more rainy days equates to less sunshine, and thus less vitamin D for the mothers of these children.

Now, on this topic, let's return to vitamin A for a moment. I was excited to receive some data from a colleague, just before this book went to press. She brought to my attention the work of Dr. Mary Megson (discussed in "New Optimum Nutrition for the Mind" by Patrick Holford; Basic Health Publications, Inc; California; 2009), a pediatrician from Virginia, who believes that autistic children are lacking in vitamin A. Being aware of the need for vitamin A to help build the lining of the digestive tract, and that Autism is often linked to the incomplete digestion of gluten (from grains) and casein (from milk), Dr. Megson speculated that vitamin A deficiency may be part of the problem. She was also well aware that the body needs vitamin A, in adequate amounts, for correct brain and vision development. It is known that the relatives of autistic children often have weak "black and white" vision. A lack of vitamin A would compound this, in ensuing generations and, since this component of vision is necessary to perceive shadow, in its absence, one would lose some of the ability to perceive in three dimensions and thus, to interpret facial expressions. Autistic children tend to look to the side instead of directly at one (considered to be a sign of poor social skills), but most of our black and white receptors occur at the edge of the visual field, so these children may just be attempting to compensate for what is missing from their visual map. Dr. Megson began giving cod liver oil to her autistic patients and reported impressive improvements, often within only weeks of beginning the treatment. In once case the patient reported "now I can see emotion on the faces on TV." And, while Dr. Megson is on track with her approach to vitamin A, we hope that she is also aware that the vitamin D in the cod liver oil is also adding to the total benefit.

CAVITIES: Again, old news, from 1934, shows that valuable information on vitamin D has been lost for some time. A study done with orphans in New York showed that as little as 1,000IU of vitamin D daily stopped cavities from forming in their teeth.

CELIAC DISEASE: As mentioned at the beginning of this chapter, there is a patent link between celiac disease and vitamin D deficiency. When we consider that vitamin A, along with vitamin D, are both required to build our internal mucosal membranes, and that they co-exist in natural food sources (in the livers of creatures that we eat), we can deduce that these two vitamins most likely work together. Add to that the massive deficiency of both A and D in the modern Western world that has been going on for decades. Since we know now that vitamin A can rebuild the cilia (fine hairs that keep the lungs clean), it is very possible that high doses of vitamins A and D may rebuild the villi (fine hairs on the intestinal tract), the absence of which is the root cause of celiac disease.

CROHN'S DISEASE: In early 2010, a study put out by McGill University Health Centre, suggested that vitamin D might prevent and fight Crohn's disease, and possibly ulcerative colitis as well. It has been observed that Crohn's disease is more common amongst people who live in the northern climates; in fact, Canada has one of the highest rates of this disease in the world. During lab experiments on cancer cells, the ensuing genetic analysis of the cells showed that vitamin D switched on two genes that have been found to be important in preventing or treating Crohn's disease. While it is indicated that clinical studies are needed to confirm this, researchers did go on to suggest that "siblings of patients with Crohn's disease that haven't yet developed the disease might be well advised to make sure they're vitamin D sufficient."

HEART DISEASE: A study printed in the journal "Circulation," showed that those men with low vitamin D levels, had a 62% increased risk of heart failure compared to those with sufficient levels. Vitamin D has been found to lower "C-reactive protein" levels in the blood, which is an early marker of heart disease potential. Pediatric cardiomyopathy (infant heart failure) was linked to chronic vitamin D deficiency, beginning with the mother.

JUVENILE DIABETES: A study done in Finland in 2001 found that if children were given 2,000IU of vitamin D daily, the risk of them developing Juvenile Diabetes was reduced by 80%.

PSORIASIS: Since psoriasis is often treated with ultraviolet light, it made me wonder if high levels of supplemental vitamin D might not have a similar effect on this skin disorder. Sure enough, my research revealed that some early studies found patients with psoriasis to have low blood levels of vitamin D. As well, applying vitamin D topically to those with psoriasis has been shown to reduce the symptoms.

SCHIZOPHRENIA: This ailment occurs 10% more often among those born in the early spring and winter, when less vitamin D from the sun is available. Studies done to test this thesis on rats, have found that when you deprive the mother rats of vitamin D, their offspring have reduced nerve growth and excessive cell proliferation. John McGrath from Queensland Brain Institute said "What we see is that when you take D out of the brain in the rodent, you can break their brain basically."

CHAPTER THREE

B VITAMINS: TOO MUCH OF A GOOD THING?

Getting back to our basic one-a-day multi-vitamin. You will find that good formulas can comfortably include about 25mg to 30mg of most of the family of B vitamins in the one pill, which is usually sufficient for the average person. The B complex should include at least 20mg of B-6, 100mcg of B-12 and 1mg of folic acid, these being the optimal amounts required to prevent the build-up of homocysteine in the blood. High homocysteine levels allow cholesterol to trap in the arteries (atherosclerosis), leading to heart disease.

If you feel the need for a higher level of B vitamins, perhaps due to high stress levels, and you decide to take an extra B-complex, take it at a separate meal from the ones you get in your one-a-day. Taking them together will only give you expensive urine, since the blood can only hold so much of the B vitamins in one sitting. The best way to take B vitamins, whether in a complex or as single B's, is in divided doses spaced throughout the day.

Even those who are not that familiar with nutritional supplements are aware that B-vitamins are good for stress. And as a general rule this is true, though of course, the functions of B-vitamins are far broader than simply helping with stress. Using single B-vitamins can be viewed as similar to amino acids. If we take them all together (which basically means as a protein) they will serve general functions in the body. But, if we use isolated, single amino acids, they will have a more specific therapeutic function. So it is with B-vitamins. A vitamin B-complex will serve your general well being, but for example, there wouldn't be enough B-3 to lower cholesterol levels. This would require 1500 mg of B-3, as either niacin or "flush-free" niacin. Let's have a brief look at some of the functions of each B-vitamin on its own.

THE INDIVIDUAL B'S

B-1: THIAMINE: Important for digestive functions, mental function and cognition; protects against damage caused by excess alcohol and tobacco. Deficiency symptoms: fatigue, loss of appetite, irritability, numbness in hands and feet, weakness and severe weight loss. Depleted by: caffeine intake, antibiotics, birth control pills, alcohol; alcohol inhibits its storage, so the most common deficiency in the West occurs amongst alcoholics.

B-2: RIBOFLAVIN: Necessary for the metabolism of fats, carbohydrates and proteins, helps build red blood cells and aids in preventing cataracts, and is required for glutathione production in the body. Along with vitamins A and D, riboflavin works to rebuild and maintain mucosal membranes. Deficiency symptom: poor digestion, dandruff, cracks and sores at the corner of the mouth, skin lesions, dermatitis, inflammation of the mouth and tongue.

B-3: NIACIN, NIACINAMIDE: Needed for healthy circulation and nervous system. Used for production of stomach acid and digestion of fats, carbohydrates and proteins. Niacin lowers cholesterol, but niacinamide does not, however, both forms of B-3 will raise serotonin levels and have been used to treat mental illness and schizophrenia. Niacin causes a flush 15 to 20 minutes after ingesting it, which lasts for about 15 minutes. One usually starts with a 100mg pill and gradually works up to tolerating a 500mg tab.

The flush is harmless and is most effective for fast improvement of circulation. Timed release is no longer considered safe, but the flush-free form of niacin works well for cholesterol. Since there is no flush, one can immediately move to the 1500mg daily required for lowering cholesterol levels. Niacin both lowers "bad" cholesterol (LDL) and raises "good" cholesterol (HDL). The niacin-flush is helpful when used before a detoxification bath, or sauna, as it brings blood to the surface of the skin facilitating the elimination of chemicals, drugs and heavy metals. Niacin can be used before sexual activity to enhance orgasm, due to its effect on histamine release (histamine is required for orgasm). Deficiency symptoms: canker sores, fatigue, loss of appetite, skin eruptions, insomnia, depression, dementia, schizophrenia, and pellagra.

B-5: PANTOTHENIC ACID: Another B-vitamin necessary for metabolism of fats, carbohydrates and proteins, this one is critical for maintaining the adrenal hormones, reducing stress and for the production of neurotransmitters. A usual dose for stress and adrenal health is 250mg three times per day. Deficiency symptoms: fatigue, headaches, nausea, anxiety, depression and tingling in the hands.

B-6: PYRIDOXINE: Required for the production of stomach acid and red blood cells. Supports the immune system, neurotransmitter function, helps prevent kidney stones (with magnesium) and prevents homocysteine build-up. Deficiency symptoms: Water retention (esp. during PMS), sore tongue, acne, cracks or sores on mouth and lips, numbness and tingling sensations, carpel tunnel syndrome, anorexia. Depleted by antidepressants, birth control pills, diuretics and estrogen replacement therapy.

B-12: METHYLCOBALAMIN: This is the new, better-absorbed form of vitamin B-12, replacing the old "cyanocobalamin" form. When taken sublingually (under the tongue) it is the closest thing to an injection of B-12. This vitamin protects the nervous system, and is currently used at high levels (40-60mg) to treat nervous system disorders like Parkinson's Disease, Bell's Palsy and multiple sclerosis. It has the potential to regenerate damaged nerves, and can prevent nerve damage caused by aging and toxins. B-12 is important for memory and learning, and prevents pernicious anemia by helping to build red blood cells. It is also necessary to prevent homocysteine build-up that can lead to arterial plaque. Deficiency can be caused by strict vegetarianism and aging; and as well certain blood types are prone to B-12 deficiency (type A and type AB). These circumstances can cause one to lose the ability to absorb this vitamin through the gut, which is why the medical profession uses injection, although the sublingual form is almost as effective as injection. Due to its critical importance for healthy aging, there will be a separate chapter on B-12. Deficiency symptoms: inflammation of the tongue, irritability, nervousness, depression, chronic fatigue, memory loss, migraines and spinal cord degeneration. Depleted by anticoagulants and anti-gout medications.

BIOTIN: Aids in fatty acid production, cell growth, and digestion of fats, carbohydrates and proteins. Required for healthy skin and hair. Deficiency symptoms: Loss of appetite, nausea, sore tongue, anemia, depression, hair loss and insomnia. Depleted by raw egg whites, rancid oils and antibiotics.

CHOLINE: Lecithin is rich in choline and often is the best way to get it therapeutically (as granules, or as Phosphatidyl Choline in capsule form). Choline is critical for nerve transmission from the brain and for gall bladder and liver function. Because it is necessary to metabolize fat and cholesterol, choline will clean fatty deposits off of the liver and out of the arteries. Deficiency symptoms: Poor fat digestion, impaired short term memory, fatty liver, high blood pressure, atherosclerosis, nervous system disorders.

FOLIC ACID: Helps with cell division and replication, energy production and red blood cell production. Supports immune function by helping to produce white blood cells. Needed to regulate homocysteine levels. Folic acid is critical before and during pregnancy to prevent the birth defect "spina bifida." In Canada, law limits supplements to one milligram of folic acid per day, which is the minimal one should have for health. This means that if you buy a multivitamin that recommends 3 pills per day (like many prenatal multi's), that milligram of folic acid is divided between the 3 pills. And if you only take one pill per day you are getting shorted on your folic acid intake. Choose a good quality "one-a-day" as it will have the whole milligram of folic acid in one pill. Deficiency symptoms: Sore, red tongue, digestive problems, anemia, apathy, graying hair, insomnia and memory problems. Depleted by oral contraceptives and alcohol (at high levels), and destroyed by cooking.

INOSITOL: A component of lecithin, along with choline, inositol also helps to metabolize fatty deposits off of the liver and out of the arteries, and aids in lowering cholesterol. It is a calming agent that is used at high dosage levels to treat depression, anxiety and Obsessive Compulsive Disorder. Deficiency symptoms: Constipation, irritability, skin eruptions, hair loss, high cholesterol and atherosclerosis.

PABA: Para-Aminobenzoic Acid helps the body to digest and utilize protein. It is needed to make red blood cells and can be converted into folic acid in the intestines. Protects the lungs against pollutants and supports healthy intestinal flora. Once commonly used in natural sun blocks to protect against sunburn and skin cancer, but since many people were apparently allergic to PABA, it is not used for that purpose much anymore. Deficiency symptoms: Grey hair, fatigue, irritability, nervousness, depression, gastrointestinal disorders and vitiligo. Depleted by antibiotics and sulfa drugs.

HOW TO USE THE B-VITS

Remember that if you want to use any single B-vitamin at a therapeutic dose level, you must also take a B-complex, though not necessarily at the same dosage level. This is because the B-vitamins are an interdependent family of nutrients. Therefore, a high dosage of one B-vitamin will eventually deplete some of the other B's. So for example, if you are taking 500mg to 1000mg of B-5 for adrenal function, be sure to get 30mg to 50mg of the other B's in a B-complex or multi-vitamin.

In fact, it is better to get your B's in a multiple vitamin and mineral formula, since B's are better absorbed in the presence of minerals. Timed release multi-vitamins and B-complex pills are less effectively absorbed because it has been found that the B-vitamins are picked-up in the upper intestinal tract, but timed release pills will eventually settle into the lower intestinal tract, reducing absorption. At this point we will address the crux of the title: "Too much of a good thing?" As usual, many people think that if some is good, more is better. So we often see people taking a 50mg B-complex a couple of times per day, or using a multi-vitamin with 25mg to 50mg of each of the B's, backed up by an additional B-complex, that usually contains 50mg of each of the B's, or more.

MEGA-DOSING AS A GOOD IDEA

Now before I explain why this is a bad idea, let me qualify: In the field of "Orthomolecular Nutrition", developed primarily by the pioneer researchers Dr. Abram Hoffer and Dr. Linus Pauling, vitamins are used in high doses as alternatives to, or to reduce the amount of, pharmaceutical drugs. Dr. Hoffer's treatment of schizophrenia and other mental disorders, with massive doses of vitamin B-3, and other nutrients, is renown worldwide.

Because certain ailments cause, or are caused by, mal-absorption of essential nutrients, very high doses can often be wonderfully effective. I've seen photos of children with Down's Syndrome who were put on a dosage of nutrients ten times what most people would take. After six months their health and mental capacity improved phenomenally and even the shape of their eyes and tongues returned to (what is considered) normal. Dixie Tafoya, who figured this out with her own child, based on the work of Dr. Henry Turket done in the 1940's, discovered that Down's Syndrome children have a metabolic malfunction that causes them to require ten times the normal amount of nutrients, that most people require to function in a healthy state. If anyone wishes to pursue this further, simply do a web search for Dixie Tafoya. One debatable aspect of her approach is the claim that the mega-doses of vitamins are hard on the livers of the children so treated. This is very possible, as you will see.

The point here is, that there is a place for mega-dosing under the care of a trained practitioner, and in cases of ill health and disease. In fact, that vitamin mega-dosing should occupy the place currently inhabited by pharmaceutical drugs. My father had epilepsy and high blood pressure in his mid-thirties. He cured both of these conditions himself, by becoming what was known in those days as a "health food nut."

MEGA-DOSING AS A BAD IDEA

Back to why the average person, in reasonably good health, shouldn't take excessive B-vitamins. First, (doing the arithmetic with a Nutritional Almanac) I estimated that it requires approximately 10 days worth of eating to get approximately 25mg of B-vitamins from food. When we take 10, 20 or more days' worth of any nutrient, especially at one meal, for extended periods, the body tends not to utilize that nutrient optimally.

The R.D.A. in America recommends 1.5mg of B-1 daily and 1.7mg of B-2. While it is acknowledged in the supplement field that these recommendations are too low, the reason they are set low is based on what food actually provides. For example:

	Vit. B-1	Vit. B-2
2 slices of whole wheat bread	.18mg	.1mg
1oz Cheddar Cheese	.11mg	.02mg
2 slices Turkey Roll	.05mg	.16mg
One Apple with skin	.02mg	.07mg
½ cup Potato Salad	.1mg	.08mg
Total	.46mg	.43mg

So, here is an example of an average lunch, totaling less than half a milligram each of vitamin B-1 and vitamin B-2. Multiply this by 5 meals (to be generous) and we are averaging less than 2.5mg of each of these two vitamins as a daily intake. Therefore, 25mg of either of these two B vitamins is basically akin to eating 10 days worth of food intake at one meal. Can we seriously advocate taking 4 times this much (100mg per day, as provided by some products, or by stacking a B complex on top of a strong multi-vitamin)? The body is simply not made to absorb huge levels of nutrients at one time, or on a consistent basis.

We are essentially, biologically, still hunter-gatherers. Our bodies are used to finding a hoard of a particular nutrient, or family of nutrients, and then not finding it again for a protracted time. Thus, the body becomes trained to conserve and utilize nutrients in the most efficient way possible. When we are too generous with these nutrients, the body believes that they are so prevalent in the environment that it need not be efficacious, because they will continue to be so commonly available that it need not be.

This principle holds true for most isolated and concentrated nutrients (vitamins, minerals and even herbs). I suggest that the easy approach is to simply skip the weekends: five days on and two days off, unless you are actively treating an ailment. Those of us who take a wide range of supplements often follow a more random pattern of use, allowing for intuition (a highly under-utilized function) to come into play. It is more valuable in this case to use supplements more casually and occasionally, than to overload our bodies and to create what I call "pill fatigue." If you are not a pill-person, don't create a lot of pressure for yourself and turn supplementing into a job, or you will just throw up your hands and give up.

Remember also to take your B's and most of the isolated nutrients (not herbs) with food. These elements exist with hundreds of other elements when found in food, and when they are synthesized or isolated to make vitamins, they are missing these co-factors necessary for their proper absorption. Here we arrive at reason number two for not taking excess B-vitamins. You may be confused hearing me talk about synthesized vitamins, believing that they are "natural". They are natural in the sense that (as someone smarter than me once said) the body recognizes vitamin B-3 (a precursor to the calming neurotransmitter serotonin) but it does not recognize Prozac (a "selective serotonin re-uptake inhibitor"). Nonetheless almost all B-vitamins are synthesized in laboratories and not isolated from foods. Let's look at a few of examples of how a B-vitamin is made.

HOW TO MAKE A B-VITAMIN

This is an example of how Vitamin B-1 is made: "Thiamine is synthesized from acetonitrile, which is derived from acetic acid (from the distillation of wood). Acetonitrile is chemically combined with ammonia forming the thiamine molecule."

Vitamin B-2: "Produced by aerobic fermentation (submerged culture with continuous agitation and aeration) using a yeast-like fungus (Eremothecium ashbyii) in a medium of D-ribose (from glucose) or various other mediums containing carbohydrates, vegetable oils and amino acids. The riboflavin is then extracted from this fermentation liquor with solvents or reducing chemicals. Riboflavin is responsible for the red-orange color of the B-complex. All yeast-like residues are removed in the extraction step."

Vitamin B-3 (Niacin): "Synthesized from acetaldehyde (from

calcium carbide and water) or pyridine (from the distillation of wood) through several chemical reactions." Vitamin B-6 (Pyridoxine Hcl): "Synthesized from the end product of the distillation of wood. Several chemical reactions involved, such as condensation, oxidation and acidification." Choline: "Synthesized from ethylene (from petroleum) and ammonia. Several chemical reactions involved using water, carbon dioxide and hydrochloric acid. The use of hydrochloric acid produces the chloride form of choline."

TOO MANY B'S

The most obvious problem with the old school approach to supplementing with vitamins is the outdated idea that you can't have too many B vitamins. It is not as simple as just having the world's most expensive urine (that bright yellow color is the excess B-2 spilling over into the urine). Excess vitamins are a burden on the liver. This is why we will find some people who get nauseous from vitamins, more so when taking vitamins on an empty stomach. So, we must appreciate that vitamin pills are not "natural," per se.

Since these are essentially pharmaceutical white powders, they are perceived by the body as chemicals and must be processed through the liver. I have seen those with liver damage unable to take mega-doses of vitamins because of the danger caused by putting additional stress on an already over-taxed liver. Thus, the important point to note is that, contrary to marketing, we need to look at vitamins as closer to drug therapy and a little less like a totally benign way of compensating for an inadequate diet.

Certainly vitamins and minerals can compensate somewhat for a decline in our quality of food (due to agribusiness practices including hybridizing plants, excessive pesticide use, synthetic fertilizers and erosion of topsoil), and poor dietary choices on our part. They must, however, be treated with care and caution. Too much zinc can deplete you of copper; too much copper can steal zinc;

too much calcium will deplete you of magnesium, etc. Unless you are doing a lot of reading and research in the field of nutrition, or utilizing trained professionals, it is best to err on the side of caution when self-prescribing vitamins and minerals; even the supposedly safest ones, the water-soluble B-vitamins.

The bottom line can be summed up in a phrase that is widely applicable to most of modern living: “More is not better.”

Next, to bring that one-a-day multivitamin up to the level where you get the amount of nutrients scientifically proven to help protect against cancer and heart disease, it is essential to add extra vitamin C (a minimum of 500mg) and vitamin E (at least 400IU).

CHAPTER FOUR

VITAMIN C: WORSE THAN SUGAR?

Is vitamin C worse than sugar? Of course not, this is what we in the writing business call a "hook." But there is truth in that statement, with regards to chewable vitamin C. Most chewable vitamin C does worse damage to the teeth than chewing on sugar cubes. This is because common vitamin C is a compound known as ascorbic acid, and that level of acidity is more corrosive to tooth enamel than sugar. Sugar is also problematic because it feeds bacteria in the mouth that can cause cavities.

Currently, the worst beverage for causing tooth decay is now believed to be commercial iced-tea products, having replaced colas, the previous worst offenders. This is because of the high amounts of citric acid added to these products in order to get a lemon-like tang; citric acid being less expensive to use than real lemon juice. Citric acid and ascorbic acid are similar in the levels of acidity they possess.

Citric acid is not bad for you, in moderation, whereas ascorbic acid is good for you, since it does function as vitamin C in the body. There is, however, a better form of vitamin C called buffered vitamin C. Buffered vitamin C (also known as pH-neutral or ascorbate) is not acidic in nature, and used in chewable form is not damaging to the teeth. Buffered vitamin C does not taste quite as good as ascorbic acid, since it tastes tart, while ascorbates tend to taste bitter.

BUFFERED VITAMIN C

Now, chewing aside, let's compare ascorbic acid to buffered vitamin C. It turns out that mammals, except for our species and one or two other creatures, manufacture their own vitamin C in their bodies, producing it in a non-acidic form. Since humans cannot manufacture vitamin C in their bodies it must obtained from our diet. Therefore, when we ingest ascorbic acid, our body must react it with a mineral in order that the ascorbic acid is efficiently utilized.

Taking a gram (1000mg) or two per day is not going to be an issue for most people (though there are some people who can't take any acidic vitamin C, without it upsetting their stomach). If you choose, however, to take high dosage levels of ascorbic acid, say 6,000mg or more, daily, you are adding to your load of acidic substances, as well as depleting the body of the minerals required to neutralize that acid load. If you are familiar with the acid/alkaline theory of health, you will appreciate that most people already ingest too many acidic substances, leaving them in an over-acidic condition, which leads to disease.

Buffered vitamin C is made by reacting ascorbic acid, which is acidic, with a mineral, which is alkaline, creating a pH-neutral ascorbate form of the vitamin. In this form it is retained in the body for at least three times longer than ascorbic acid, which washes out of the blood in about two hours. The most common form is calcium ascorbate, but some companies do mixed mineral ascorbates. This is of advantage if you want to take high dosage levels of buffered vitamin C, but do not wish to get too high a level of calcium, which is often already too high in many people, due to an excessive intake of dairy products. Multi-mineral ascorbates include magnesium ascorbate, potassium ascorbate, zinc ascorbate, etc.

The other problem with high doses of ascorbic acid is that it can cause a laxative effect. This can be a safe way to obtain such an effect, if one requires a laxative. In past decades, when ascorbic acid was pretty much the only vitamin C option, it was suggested by pioneer in the field of nutrition and godfather of vitamin C, Dr. Linus Pauling, that one consistently increase the dose of ascorbic acid until hitting "bowel tolerance." At that point reduce the intake to a level just below the laxative effect. It was believed that this indicated your optimal therapeutic vitamin C intake. Interestingly, Dr. Pauling also maintained that people born prematurely can take so much vitamin C that they seldom hit the bowel tolerance level.

BIOFLAVONOIDS

Like all nutrients, vitamin C does not exist in isolation in nature. The most important co-factors for vitamin C are bioflavonoids. When I was a kid we would often eat the peel of the orange as well as the fruit, and the white of the orange or grapefruit is where the bioflavonoids exist. Kids, please don't try this at home, unless your citrus fruit is organic. Non-organic citrus fruit has a number of nasty chemicals on the peel including pesticides, coloring agents and waxes.

Bioflavonoids work synergistically with vitamin C, each enhancing the assimilation of the other. Aside from them both functioning as antioxidants, both serve to support connective tissues, and a deficiency of both can show up as bruising too easily. Flavonoids especially, keep the veins and capillaries strong, preventing spider lines, varicose veins and hemorrhoids, and serve to promote circulation. The effectiveness of inexpensive "citrus bioflavonoids" is debatable. These can be just citrus pulp waste, with little or no biological activity.

Look instead for quality bioflavonoids (those with proven activity in the body), including rutin and hesperidin, or, for more powerful anti-inflammatory effects, quercetin, which can also help control symptoms of asthma and allergies. Two other powerful forms of bioflavonoids, for those in need of therapeutic doses (i.e. for varicose veins) are grape seed extract and Pycnogenol (a patented product derived from pine bark).

HOW MUCH?

We all know that vitamin C helps to prevent colds and, of course, scurvy. But vitamin C is also used in hundreds of metabolic functions in the body. Based on reams of scientific studies, I would say that if you were to choose only one nutrient to supplement with, vitamin C would be the most important and probably the most value for your dollar, as well.

For optimal health your intake of vitamin C should be at least 500mg three times daily. While one may take much more vitamin C quite safely, 500mg is the minimal dose required to elevate glutathione levels, thus enhancing immune and detoxification functions in the body. Increasing the dosage, however, above 500mg, while it may have other benefits, such as fighting infection and preventing heart disease, will not elevate glutathione any more than 500mg will. So, when using vitamin C at moderate levels, it is best to take it in divided doses throughout the day, especially since it is a water-soluble nutrient (and not stored for long periods, unlike fat-soluble nutrients and minerals). Either form of vitamin C will work for this purpose.

Iron absorption is greatly increased when vitamin C is taken with a meal. Also, if you have a meal high in saturated fats, such as a burger and a milkshake, as little as 500mg will prevent the thickening of the blood that then occurs. Therefore, I will make a point of taking vitamin C with any high fat meal. Higher doses may not elevate immune function much more, but it can have other therapeutic effects. For example, 6 to 12 grams, divided throughout the day, can fight most forms of infection in the body from colds and bladder infection, to abscess and prostatitis. Dr. Pauling himself took 18 grams daily, maintaining that most mammals near to our bodyweight would produce at least 10 to 12 grams per day.

HEART DISEASE

Dr. Pauling lived to 92 years of age, though truth be told, he also took one baby aspirin and a shot of vodka per day in his later years. Both of these prevent platelet clumping in the blood, helping to stop heart disease. Vitamin C also has a role to play here. It reduces LDL, or bad cholesterol, and elevates HDL, good cholesterol. In fact, some researchers believe that heart disease is simply a form of advanced scurvy, or vitamin C deficiency.

Symptoms of scurvy, or extreme vitamin C deficiency, are fatigue, bleeding and bruising easily, weakening of blood vessels, and hair and tooth loss. Since vitamin C helps synthesize collagen, the structural component of blood vessels, as well as tendons and ligaments, we can see that a decline in the protective qualities offered to blood vessels, veins and capillaries could be related to arteriosclerosis (which is a general hardening of the arteries, as opposed to atherosclerosis which is a hardening and narrowing of the arteries due to calcification and plaque build-up).

Remember that the R.D.A (Recommended Daily Allowance) of a vitamin is only the level at which a nutrient is required to inhibit disease. Therefore, the current R.D.A. of 75mg (for men) to 90mg (for women) of vitamin C, for adults, will prevent scurvy from manifesting but it will not necessarily be the ideal amount for optimal health and longevity. Sad to say, a study done at the University of Toronto in 2009 found one in seven young Canadian adults to have a deficient level of vitamin C, while 33 per cent had sub-optimal levels. I say sad, because of course, their benchmark was the above- mentioned low R.D.A levels.

So, how much vitamin C to take? Well, that is a personal decision based on your health and your intake of fresh fruits and vegetables. Can we get enough vitamin C from fresh fruits and vegetables? Perhaps, if you live in the tropics and can consume fresh fruit. But, I have seen a pH test done on a juicy orange that showed it had no vitamin C in it at all, because it had been in cold storage for nearly a year (like many fruits and vegetable are now stored).

Many studies on long-term supplementation with vitamin C (either form) have shown positive benefits: 250mg to one gram daily reduced the occurrence of the common cold by 50%; 500mg daily improved blood vessel dilation, helping to treat angina, hypertension, arteriosclerosis and congestive heart failure; in an overview of over 200,000 adults followed for 10years, a minimum of 700mg of vitamin C daily reduced the risk of coronary heart disease by 25%. Other studies have shown a lower risk of cancer of the breast, lung and stomach, and a lower incident of cataracts, at even lower dosage levels. Certain clinics give vitamin C intravenously at doses up to 70 grams per day to treat cancer, alcoholism and heroin addiction

WARNINGS

Studies have indicated that up to 10 grams of vitamin C could be taken daily with no fear of toxicity or any damage to ones' health. Yet, as you recall from the chapter on B-vitamins, any consistent excessive intake of isolated nutrients can lead to the body using it less effectively. This has been shown to be especially true with vitamin C. The person who takes 15 grams daily will be more prone to showing signs of scurvy faster when they are no longer able to acquire that amount, or stop ingesting vitamin C at that level.

Whereas, those on a more reasonable dose, of say 2 or 3 grams per day, will not have this effect, known as "rebound scurvy." Pregnant women should generally take no more than 5 grams daily or the infant could become dependent, and also develop scurvy too easily. Aside from damage to tooth enamel from chewing ascorbic acid tablets, the only other concern would be if one has too much iron in the blood, since vitamin C increases iron absorption from food up to 40%.

Certain drugs, including anti-depressants and oral contraceptives, alcohol and especially tobacco smoke, deplete vitamin C from the body.

CHAPTER FIVE

VITAMIN E: IT'S NOT JUST ALPHA ANYMORE

Returning to our hypothetical one-a-day multivitamin, you will find that, due to its limited size, it will only be able to provide from 50IU to 150IU of vitamin E. As mentioned earlier, the multivitamin provides insufficient vitamin E for most people, unless you have close to an ideal diet (5 –7 servings of fruits and vegetables daily, and plenty of whole grains, seeds, and nuts).

Vitamin E is one of the best researched essential nutrients and is part of the family of antioxidants that is critical for preventing cancer, heart disease and premature aging, by fighting the damaging free radicals produced as a byproduct of oxidation. This family is known as ACES because it includes vitamin A (as natural beta carotene), vitamin C, vitamin E and the mineral Selenium.

ACES

Selenium is a trace mineral commonly deficient in the modern diet, and distinctly linked to preventing breast and prostate cancer, as well as being a powerful anti-viral agent. Vitamin E and selenium work together to amplify each other's attributes, and due to this synergistic relationship they should be taken in tandem. Supplemental levels of selenium range from 100mcg to 200mcg daily, although higher levels are often prescribed for those with viral conditions, or cancer. Most of the research has been done on yeast-derived selenium, and while there are new fancier versions of this mineral, the yeast form is still the best bang for your buck.

The ACES are the nutritional antioxidants, which also serve countless other important functions in the body. There are many other supplemental forms of antioxidants derived from foods, such as extracts of berries, grape seed, green tea and turmeric, to name but a few, but these, even though they may be more powerful than the ACES, do not serve essential nutritional functions. Therefore, the ACES should be the base platform of our antioxidant program, before we start adding the more obscure ones, many often riding in on the latest marketing hype.

FUNCTIONS OF VITAMIN E

First identified in 1936, vitamin E has been shown to be an important fertility nutrient in the diet of rats. The name "tocopherol" was chosen from two Greek words that mean "birth" and "carry", in other words it means "to carry a pregnancy", so its first observed effects were on healthy fertility.

Aside from being an antioxidant, Vitamin E oxygenates tissue, improves circulation and supports immune functions (in part by protecting the thymus gland). It is prescribed mainly to protect against cancer, heart disease and strokes. Vitamin E (in combination with selenium) is especially protective against the development of breast and prostate cancers.

Regular doses of vitamin E clearly protected, women at least, against blood clots by reducing their occurrence by 21% (American Heart Association Journal, Sept. 2007).

This long-term study of almost 100,000 nurses indicated a 30% lower rate of heart disease amongst those with the highest intake of vitamin E (from diet and supplement). They averaged about 200IU daily intake. Another population study done in Finland in 1994 tracked over 5,000 citizens, and concluded that there was a decreased mortality from heart disease within the group with the highest intake of vitamin E.

Other studies have indicated that this protection may only hold true for people not in the highest risk categories for stroke and heart disease. It is no surprise that one supplement would not work effectively on its own. Anyone in the danger zone for stroke and heart disease would need a comprehensive arsenal of nutritional protection, including, but not limited to, vitamin E.

A seldom-mentioned fact about antioxidant supplements is that they can have some pro-oxidant effects as well. One reason that studies often surface which seem to indicate that a given vitamin is counter-productive to health is because these nutrients are studied in isolation (especially in a petri dish or animal studies). Under these unnatural conditions, negative effects are often observed.

To counter-act this pro-oxidant tendency, we need to take antioxidants in combination, so that they each keep the others' negative aspects in check. (As we saw in the chapter on Vitamin A, the Finnish men that received both beta- carotene and vitamin E, did not show the increase in cancer rates, that those who took only synthetic beta-carotene alone did. Because beta-carotene is especially susceptible to oxidative damage, other antioxidants needed to be present to prevent this degeneration of the beta-carotene from occurring.) And, of course, when found in food, all antioxidants are in combination with a host of other nutrients and other antioxidants.

People with higher levels of vitamin E in their diet were found to have a lowered risk of getting Parkinson's disease, though supplementation was not shown to slow the progression of those already with the disease (The Lancet Neurology, May 2005). In both healthy subjects and diabetics, obvious improvements in glucose metabolism and insulin efficiency were observed (American Journal of Clinical Nutrition #61).

Other aliments also have respectable amounts of research to

support the benefits of supplementing with vitamin E. For example, in combination with vitamin C and zinc, vitamin E has been shown to help protect against age-related macular degeneration and glaucoma. As well, it has been used to treat Fibrocystic Breast Disease (600IU daily; Iodine is also needed for this condition.); Menopausal symptoms (800IU daily until symptoms reduce, then 400IU); and Tardive Dyskinesia (1600IU daily).

IS IT SAFE?

Occasionally negative media attention will make people hesitant to take vitamin E as a supplement. Inevitably these "studies" turn out to be flawed when closely analyzed. The "Shute Institute" has studied vitamin E for over 50 years and has produced countless studies supporting the ability of this nutrient to protect us against cancer and heart disease, and to enhance immune function.

Doctors Wilfred and Evan Shute ultimately did research on the effects of vitamin E on more than 30,000 subjects. In addition to proving value as an antioxidant that improves the ability of tissues to use oxygen, they concluded that vitamin E had a variety of other important functions. These include: vitamin E prevents emboli from developing from clots (which cause strokes) and reduces the development of clots; it is a vasodilator of the capillaries (small blood vessels) and heals damaged capillaries; it can reduce scar tissue; it improves muscle power in athletes and animal studies and it is useful for treating PMS.

Vitamin E has been used clinically to manage thrombosis, gangrene, ulcers, thermal and radiation burns and rheumatic fever; it protects against environmental pollution, even reducing lipid peroxidation in smokers. Also, vitamin E has shown special value in reducing ischemia (deficient blood supply) caused by myocardial infarction, renal failure and stroke.

Now, in this case, we are talking about naturally derived vitamin E, not a chemically synthesized vitamin product. Unlike the

B vitamins, which are all synthesized, vitamin E is commonly produced in two forms; the synthetic, found more commonly in pharmacies, and the natural form, dominating in the natural health field.

When purchasing vitamin E, the difference between synthetic versus natural, can be determined by carefully looking at the ingredient panel on the side of the bottle. Naturally derived vitamin E is referred to as D-Alpha Tocopherol, while synthetic vitamin E, derived from petroleum, will have an "L" after the D, and will read as "DL" (or "dl") Alpha Tocopherol. In the natural health field, it is considered to be important to choose natural vitamin E for two main reasons. One, it is more bio-available, and two, it is believed that synthetic E can block the E-receptors in the body, making it difficult to assimilate authentic vitamin E thereafter.

OTHER MEMBERS OF THE E-FAMILY

The latest developments in vitamin E research have revealed that, in fact, it is a family of nutrients, not just one. Yet, legally, only Alpha Tocopherol can be referred to as "vitamin E", even though there are eight components to the family of E.

This "family" of components that make up vitamin E include 4 tocopherols, which are known as "mixed" vitamin E (Alpha, Beta, Gamma and Delta tocopherol) and 4 tocotrienols (also Alpha, Beta, Gamma and Delta, tocotrienols).

The tocotrienols are the most powerful of the antioxidants in the family of E constituents, and are also more powerful therapeutic agents when treating cancer and heart disease. They are also considerably more expensive and less commonly available than the tocopherols, which will be our focus here.

A problem with taking high amounts (800IU and up) of only Alpha Tocopherol for long periods of time appears to be, that it can deplete the other tocopherols in the body, especially Gamma Tocopherol. Lower levels of Gamma Tocopherol have been linked to higher incidents of both breast and prostate cancers. Again, the situation is much the same as can occur with the B-vitamins; if we take high levels of only one B vitamin, for extended periods, we will eventually deplete the body of other of the B's. This is because they are an interdependent family of nutrients that are found together in food, and rely upon each other for assimilation.

Fortunately, those of us who eat a healthy diet don't really have this concern, since the family of mixed tocopherols is readily available from whole grains, seeds and nuts. Other rich sources of vitamin E in the diet include vegetable oils (especially almond, olive and sunflower), peanut butter and wheat germ. Since my diet has always (during my adult life) included plenty of these foods, I am still comfortable taking a basic naturally derived vitamin E product (Alpha Tocopherol.) Again, because there are countless scientific studies that support the use of 400IU to 1200IU of Alpha Tocopherol for a variety of health benefits.

Dr. Andrew Weil, one of the most respected voices in the alternative health field, suggests that those under the age of 40 need 400IU daily, and those over the age of 40 should have around 800IU per day.

SYMPTOMS OF DEFICIENCY

Severe vitamin E deficiency can manifest as a collection of nasty symptoms including poor coordination, involuntary eye movement, hemolytic anemia, nerve damage and muscle weakness. Those at greatest risk generally have health issues that impede fat absorption, like celiac disease, cystic fibrosis, or a missing gallbladder (those without a gallbladder can use "Bile Salts," to improve fat digestion and absorption). The dry form of vitamin E (succinate) is definitely better for those who do not digest fats well, and some studies have indicated that it is a superior antioxidant to the common oil-based form.

WARNINGS

Levels above 800IU of vitamin E have the potential to interact with blood thinning medications and can increase the anti-coagulation effect caused by vitamin K deficiency. Those with heart failure, due to hypertension or rheumatic heart disease, must start at a very low dose and gradually increase the dose until hitting 800 to 1200IU. This is because the increased strength of the heartbeat can cause problems with the weakened heart muscle. In such cases one should seek the advice of a qualified health professional before proceeding.

TOPICAL USE

Vitamin E is also often used externally to speed healing and prevent scarring. The important thing to know, when using vitamin E topically, is that it is only applied after the scab has fallen off, and fresh pink skin is revealed. At this point, the most effective treatment is to alternate applying vitamin E to the healing tissue with a comfrey ointment or cream. Comfrey can generate new cell growth in the skin, but as with vitamin E, neither must be used before the skin has healed completely. The danger lies in healing the external part of the wound before all risk of infection has been removed, so that any infection present is not trapped below the skin.

When there is no longer any indication of infection, such as inflammation radiating out from the wound area, or an angry red area that hurts, we can then begin to alternate vitamin E and comfrey topically, thereby reducing scarring to a minimum. Each substance must be applied at least twice daily, at separate times, and rubbed well into the tissue. When choosing a vitamin E for this purpose purchase natural E-400IU capsules (doesn't have to be "mixed" E) and pop them open with a pin to apply capsule contents. Most liquid vitamin E is either synthetic (but not labeled as such in the cosmetic department) or is diluted with other oils, and is not sufficiently strong enough for our purposes here.

CHAPTER SIX

DEATH BY CALCIUM

MINERALS

As far as minerals go, a good quality one-a-day should provide enough zinc (10 to 15mg) for women and young men. For older men, and/or those with prostate problems, more zinc is usually required (20mg for maintenance up to 50mg for those with prostate infections), and will be found in a gender and age specific version. Always take supplements containing zinc with food, as they can cause nausea when taken on an empty stomach. This also applies to zinc-lozenges used to treat a sore throat and cold. (Certain exceptions exist, including the trademarked supplement "ZMA" which is taken before bed by athletes, for improved sleep patterns and tissue repair; this product uses a unique form of zinc that does not cause nausea on an empty stomach.)

An interesting phenomenon about zinc in lozenge, or liquid form, is that the body cannot taste zinc when the body is deficient in zinc. But, as soon as the deficiency is satiated, the metallic, acidic or astringent qualities of the zinc can be tasted. Adding up lozenges (counting the milligrams), until the zinc can be tasted is one way to determine the body's zinc requirements. Zinc deficiency has also been linked to anorexia, due to its requirement for proper smelling and tasting functions in the body (appetite depends, in part, on fragrance and flavor). Another sign of zinc deficiency is white spots on the fingernails.

The important trace minerals should be available at reasonable levels in a multivitamin (100mcg to 200mcg of each) since they do not occupy very much space in a "one-a-day." They are called "trace" minerals because they are taken at microgram levels rather than milligram amounts. (Minerals essential to well being at microgram levels become "heavy metals" at milligram levels, and can be dangerous.) The most important trace minerals are chromium, required for maintaining stable blood sugar levels (100mcg to 200mcg), selenium, mentioned in the chapter on vitamin E (100mcg to 200mcg) and iodine, necessary for proper thyroid function (100mcg to 150mcg). Iodine probably is required at much higher levels than what is recommended in North America, but that is a subject for another book.

For older women, and those with a poor diet, the addition of extra calcium and magnesium offers protection against hypertension and osteoporosis. The amount of these two nutrients required for such purposes will not be available in a one-a-day, due to a lack of space. Also, due to lack of space, we will be focusing on calcium and magnesium in this chapter. This is because calcium is the most commonly prescribed and recommended mineral, and also the one with the most dangerous side effects, though few seem to be aware of this.

KILLING WITH CALCIUM

As mentioned before, Western thought tends to the approach that "if a little is good, a lot must be better, right"? How else to explain the medical profession instructing people (women mostly) to take 1200, 1500 and even 2000 mg of elemental calcium per day. Even the medical profession will acknowledge that all the calcium in the world will not rebuild bone-mass, but at best, simply forbid further withdrawal from the bones. Yet, they continue to promote absurd amounts of calcium with little real evidence to support their position, and in the face of recent studies that suggest that huge amounts of calcium are, in fact, dangerous. As well, what the medical profession does offer to rebuild the bone mass has proven to be dangerous.

A study from New Zealand released in 2008 has linked calcium supplementation in post-menopausal women to stroke and heart disease. The same news release included findings from the Canadian Journal of Rheumatology, which warned that using drugs designed to prevent and treat osteoporosis and fractures can cause bone tissue to collapse. "The results of our study demonstrate that bisphosphonate (also called diphosphonates, eg. "Fosamax") use is associated with an increased risk of bone necrosis..." Which means, "bone death".

In my practice I have talked with dental workers who claim that they are seeing older women with teeth that are very hard on the outside, but weak and collapsing on the inside, due to being on bisphosphonates. Here is a quotation from the Stony Brook School of Dental Medicine: "In 2003 and 2004, the first reports of patients who developed necrosis of the jawbones while taking biophosphonates (bisphosphonates) appeared in the literature...Since then, more than 500 cases have been identified and the number of these cases continues to grow" (Dent Clin North Am. 2008 Jan). Canadian physicians dispensed nearly 8 million prescriptions for bisphosphonates in 2007.

Why do doctors recommend such high levels of calcium? Well, it all started in the 50's and 60's when studies were done using calcium carbonate without any co-factors. Now, doctors have finally allowed that vitamin D might be important, but they have yet to clue into the relationship between calcium and magnesium. Since original referenced studies utilized the most difficult calcium to digest (carbonate), given on an empty stomach, in a tablet, without magnesium, let alone other co-factors such as zinc and potassium, doctors needed to get subjects to consume huge amounts of calcium before they could register any noticeable benefits. The early studies were based on upping the dosage of calcium until spillover appears in the urine; not the smartest way to determine one's need for a nutrient.

MAGNESIUM

For those who consume plenty of dairy (milk) products, it is more important to make sure that they are getting enough magnesium, rather than calcium. (I will not get into the argument that all dairy products are debatable sources of calcium anyways, since they are too high in protein and phosphorus. These elements, in excess, cause acidity in the body, further leaching minerals from the bones.) Dairy products provide too much calcium, which ultimately can deplete magnesium from the body. In traditional cultures (Asian and African) that show few signs of osteoporosis, the average daily calcium intake is far below what is recommended in the Western nations.

In fact, a recent study gave post-menopausal women only magnesium, and no calcium, and magnesium alone was enough to halt bone-loss. This response was due to the dietary situation in the West, where most people are consuming dairy products and getting plenty of calcium, but not eating sufficient amounts of dark green vegetables (broccoli, kale, chard, etc) in order to get enough magnesium into the diet to properly balance the high calcium intake.

Now that there has been a link established between calcium supplementation and increased levels of stroke and heart disease in post-menopausal women, it is time to roll back the recommended amounts of calcium. Following is a quick summary of that study, in case you wish to do more research on the subject yourself. From the Department of Medicine at the University of Auckland, New Zealand, here is their objective: "To determine the effect of calcium supplementation on myocardial infarction, stroke, and sudden death in healthy postmenopausal women." This was a "randomized, placebo controlled trial", which is considered to be of the highest scientific caliber. Their conclusion was: "Calcium supplementation in healthy postmenopausal women is associated with upward trends in cardiovascular event rates. This potentially detrimental effect should be balanced against the likely benefits of calcium on bone." (BMJ. 2008 Feb 2; Epub. 2008 Jan 15)

This link is due to depletion of magnesium by excessive calcium levels. This skewed ratio is what put those menopausal women in that New Zealand study into heart disease territory, since the heart depends on magnesium to beat regularly. Thus, an irregular heart beat, or "flutter", can usually be rectified by simply increasing one's magnesium intake, and rolling back excessive calcium intake. Another common symptom of low magnesium levels is muscle cramps ("Charlie horses"). So what happens when you go to the average doctor and tell him you have muscle cramps? You are sent off to buy calcium. The fact is: calcium contracts and constricts, and magnesium relaxes and dilates.

Magnesium sulfate for example (Epsom salts), is used in a bath to relax muscles. (By the way, an Epsom salt bath is considered a good way to raise blood levels of magnesium, if you use at least 2 cups in a hot bath.) If you have high blood pressure (the link to stroke in the study) a doctor may put you on a "calcium-channel-blocker" instead of just taking you off of calcium (which constricts blood vessels) supplements and dairy products, and giving you magnesium (which dilates and opens the blood vessels). Other symptoms of magnesium deficiency include fatigue and sleep disorders.

The other problem with excessive calcium intake is the tendency of the body to deposit it in the joints, creating arthritic conditions and bone spurs. As well, excess calcium can be deposited in soft tissue potentially leading to arteriosclerosis, glaucoma and kidney stones. If anyone has calcification anywhere in the body, the natural treatment is to stop ingesting calcium as a supplement, and from dairy products, and to simply take 500 to 600mg of magnesium per day (as citrate, in divided doses) for a few months, until the magnesium has emulsified the calcium deposits down to a level that eliminates the symptoms. (This process can be aided by using herbs containing "saponins," as explained in Part Two, Chapter Six: "Controlling Inflammation.")

CALCIUM SUPPLEMENTS

Calcium supplements are available in a variety of forms including chelate, citrate, coral and carbonate, among others. While the citrate form of calcium is usually touted at the most digestible, and the carbonate form the least, it turns out that the advantage of citrate over carbonate is only based on being taken on an empty stomach. This approach is now commonly advised by doctors, who suggest that calcium is best taken before bed. And it is true that calcium absorbs better in the evening than the day, so if you only take it once a day, suppertime would be the best.

Carbonate forms of calcium require a higher stomach acid level that is present when one is eating (especially when protein is present in the meal). "When...consumed with a meal in a person with normal stomach acid secretion, most calcium sources appear to be roughly equivalent to one another, and just about the same as from food sources." (The Nutrition Desk Reference, Robert Garrison & Elizabeth Somer, Keats Publishing, 1995, p244; Miller J, Smith D, Flora L, et al: Calcium absorption from calcium carbonate and a new form of calcium (Calcium Citrate-Malate) in healthy male and female adolescents. Am J Clin N 1988:48:1291-1294.)

And, at this juncture, let us put to bed the old myth that "Tums" are a reasonable source of calcium. Since the calcium found in Tums is in carbonate form, and the function of the tablet is to neutralize stomach acid, clearly we won't be absorbing the calcium present. (See below, under "Further Evidence.")

Citrates, like chelates, are in essence pre-digested and so do not require much stomach acid in order to be digestible. Since it is generally not advisable to take isolated nutrients on an empty stomach, if you are taking your minerals with food, the form of mineral is not that important. Some chelates are superior to others, however, with the Albion trademark being one of the few forms that is clinically tested and patented. Other highly absorbable forms of calcium available include citrate-malate and MCHC (microcrystalline hydroxyapatite, derived from young cow bones).

Daily intake of calcium, including diet, should be not much more than 500mg to 600mg of elemental calcium. Elemental refers to the actual amount of calcium absorbed. For example 1000mg of calcium citrate will provide only 200mg of actual calcium, the rest being the carrying agent: citrate. Calcium carbonate (which includes coral calcium, though coral has the advantage of also containing a wide range of trace minerals) is 40% elemental calcium, meaning that 1000mg of this form will provide 400mg of useable calcium. This also means that a product can get more elemental calcium into a smaller space, if they use a carbonate form.

Most labels are now required to state the elemental amount of minerals on the label. In Canada, when the form of mineral is in brackets then the following number must be an elemental figure. Thus: Calcium (citrate)....200mg, means that you are getting 200mg of fully utilizable calcium. Whereas: Calcium citrate... 200mg means that you are only getting 40mg of elemental calcium. This becomes a concern mostly with capsulated calcium products, which can only hold about half as much material as a tablet, and so the consumer can be confused into thinking there is more calcium present than there actually is.

The problem with tablets is that they are often poorly digested, since they are essentially little rocks (being made of compressed minerals). It is preferable to get calcium in a capsule, chewable or liquid form to guarantee digestion. One trick to test out the digestibility of a calcium pill, or any other tablet, is to put it into vinegar for an hour, then swirl it about and see if it has dissolved at all. This mimics your stomach acid and indicates the "disintegration" factor of the tablet: that is, if it breaks up in the gut or passes through, undigested.

HOW MUCH?

Every 2 parts of calcium "uses up" approximately one part of magnesium. Thus, most cal-mag products are in a 2 to 1 ratio (e.g. 300mg calcium to 150mg magnesium). This is fine for those who don't use dairy products, but for those who do use dairy on a regular basis (almost daily), I feel it is more important to pay attention to their magnesium intake. For the average dairy consumer, I will suggest a one to one ratio of calcium to magnesium, ideally about 400mg to 600mg of each, depending on age.

If you are happy taking 600mg or less of elemental calcium daily (and by "happy" I mean that you believe me and other knowledgeable consultants in the supplement field, over your doctor), you can use a one-to-one ratio of calcium to magnesium. At levels much above 600mg per day of calcium you must use the traditional two-to-one ratio, as high levels of magnesium can have a laxative effect. (Magnesium, in the inexpensive oxide form, is a good safe laxative if that is what one requires: about 500 mg, elemental, before bed. If that does not work, try 250mg at dinner and 500mg before bed.)

The advantage of taking an equal ratio cal-mag supplement is that the calcium will use half the magnesium to assimilate itself, and the other half will be available to serve other functions in the body, including helping to absorb the calcium from dairy products more efficiently. Remember that the body cannot absorb more than a maximum of 500mg of elemental calcium in one sitting, and anything more than 300mg of elemental magnesium at one serving may cause the aforementioned laxative effect. Thus, like with the B-vitamins, larger quantities must be taken in divided doses, throughout the day.

Now, why would we be satisfied with only 600mg or less, of calcium per day? Well, the historical average intake of a human in a traditional diet is from 350 to 500mg per day. These are cultures that rarely show signs of osteoporosis. Yet, we in the West get more calcium than at any other place or time in history, and have more osteoporosis, and dental decay, than any of these so called "primitive" societies. Consider it a loose conspiracy of bad science and dairy-board propaganda. (That lady dressed up as a talking cow is right there at the first grade, explaining to the children how ice cream is a good source of calcium.)

REBUILDING BONE MASS

So, instead of overloading the system with too much of one element, calcium, we will add substances that are powerful co-factors in the absorption of calcium; items that will channel the calcium back into the bone mass and contribute to rebuilding it. The three best-researched substances are the trace minerals boron and silica along with vitamin K2.

Silica is available in a few different forms, but currently I would recommend it in the form of aqueous extract of horsetail, for the purposes of bone rebuilding (3 to 6 capsules per day). Other valid forms of supplemental silica include colloidal gel, orthosilic acid and bamboo-derived silica. In Europe, doctors will more commonly prescribe silica supplementation for healing broken bones, rather than calcium. It is important to note that bones require more than just the hardness factor that calcium provides. They also need to be flexible enough to absorb a shock without snapping. That is what silica brings to the equation. Silica also keeps your arteries flexible, your skin elastic, and strengthens your hair, teeth and nails.

Boron, aside from increasing bone density, has also been used to treat arthritis. It has been shown to protect against prostate cancer, and may have benefit in regulating estrogen in women and testosterone in men (3mg per day is the usual dosage of boron). It has been observed by researchers that many people with osteoporosis have an impaired ability to convert inactive vitamin D, in the body, into its most biologically active form (a variation of D3). It is now believed that boron is important to this conversion process; all the more necessary, because of the widespread vitamin D deficiency in the West, that we have just discussed.

Vitamin K2, known for its clotting ability on the blood, has been used for decades in Japan to treat osteoporosis, and has proved to be important to preventing calcium deposition in the arteries. Unfortunately, it has until recently been restricted as a supplement in Canada, even though it is now known vitamin K deficiency is widespread, due mostly to the fact that we feed our cattle and cows grain, instead of grasses. Grass-fed cows provide vitamin K2 in the milk and grass-fed cattle provide it in the meat. Some vitamin K is also found in organ meats and egg yolks.

Vitamin K2 comes in two forms known as MK4 and MK7 and both have science substantiating them. Because vitamin K2, however, is restricted in Canada to microgram servings, and MK4 appears to only work in milligram amounts, the Canadian is advised to choose the MK7 form, which can be effective at 120micrograms.

A study published in the American Journal of Clinical Nutrition (Jan. 1999) was designed to compare vitamin K intake and hip fractures in women. This study concluded: "Low intakes of vitamin K may increase the risk of hip fracture in women. The data support the suggestion for a reassessment of the vitamin K requirements that are based on bone health and blood coagulation." One interesting point in this study was that the "risk of hip fracture was also inversely associated with lettuce consumption (…for one or more servings per day compared with one or fewer serving per week), the food that contributed the most to dietary vitamin K intakes." This is because vitamin K1 is found in leafy, green vegetables and, while not as valuable for bone density as K2, clearly does provide some benefit in this department. One obvious sign of vitamin K deficiency is tendency to easy bruising. If such a symptom does not respond to increased levels of vitamin C and bioflavonoids, the easy bruising may then be due to vitamin K deficiency.

When we see how these co-factors can help absorb the macrominerals, it becomes obvious how ridiculous it is to suggest, as many doctors do, that you take your isolated calcium, maybe with vitamin D, on an empty stomach, before bed. Calcium in food will exist with countless other elements (there are 70 to 90 trace minerals found in topsoil), and if we know that magnesium, vitamin D, vitamin K2, zinc, potassium, silica and boron, all improve the assimilation of calcium, then it stands to reason that many other dietary factors may also be important to fully absorb and utilize this important mineral. So take your calcium with a meal.

If I've offended you or your doctor, I'm sorry, and really it's not their fault. The medical associations prevent doctors from even talking about supplementation or alternative treatments, and premeds spend very little time studying nutrition in medical school. But, when we look at the health crisis facing North America as the boomers age, en mass, it is apparent that the obvious solution is an integrated medical system that encourages both alternative and preventative health care.

FURTHER EVIDENCE

"Don't count on milk to beat osteoporosis. In a Harvard study of 78,000 nurses (The Harvard Nurse's Study; Cumming & Klineberg; American Journal of Epidemiology) drinking 3 or more glasses of milk per day did not reduce fractures at all. An Australian study (Australian Study; Feskanich; American Journal of Public Health) showed the same thing." – Physician's Committee for Responsible Health

"Current use of calcium supplements was associated with increased risk of hip...and vertebral...fractures; current use of Tums antacid tablets was associated with increased risk of fractures of the proximal humerus…In conclusion, this study did not find a substantial beneficial effect of calcium on fracture risk." – Cumming, et al; "Calcium intake and fracture risk: results from the study of osteoporotic fractures"; American Journal of Epidemiology, 1997.

"The more calcium people consumed, the more susceptible they seemed to be to hip fractures. People in those countries that consume the highest levels of dairy foods (North America and Northern European nations) take in two or three times more calcium yet break two or three times more bones than people with the lowest calcium intake (Asians and African)…Most Chinese were getting their calcium from vegetables and fruits alone. Although they got less than half the calcium recommended by the USDA, their bones seemed healthy. Among women over 50, the hip fracture rate appeared to be one fifth as high as Western nations." – Discover Magazine, Aug. 2000; Dr. Colin Campbell, Cornell University (Author of "The China Study").

CHAPTER SEVEN

WHICH ESSENTIAL FATTY ACID IS FOR YOU?

Essential fatty acids are an important part of a complete supplement program. A multivitamin will not contain fatty acids, as they generally must be in a liquid form (although that liquid may be found in a "softgel" capsule).

Essential fatty acids are defined as such since they must be obtained from the diet (thus are "essential") and cannot be produced in the body from other elements. They are required for a wide range of functions including regulation of metabolism and maintenance of reproductive functions. As well EFA's are needed for early growth and development, for normal brain function, bone health and stimulation of hair and skin growth.

OMEGA 3

Most people are already aware that they should be supplementing with Omega 3 fatty acids. We have heard and read enough about how fish oils prevent heart disease and are important for mental health, healthy skin and are needed to keep inflammatory conditions in check. There is, however, some confusion on which fish oil to choose and whether or not flax oil is a viable alternative to fish oil. The confusion arises with fish oils from the fact that all the capsules are the same size (usually 1000mg to 1200mg) yet contain varying amounts of Omega 3's. Remember that, for general preventative purposes, we should obtain approximately 1000mg of Omega 3's daily (much more for therapeutic purposes).

To explain in more detail, let's look at the level of the two prime components that make up Omega 3 Fatty Acids: DHA (Docosahexaenoic Acid) and EPA (Eicosapentaenoic Acid). A capsule of Pacific salmon oil contains about 80mg of EPA and 70mg of DHA (Arctic salmon can provide up to 200mg of total omega 3s and some salmon oil caps are fortified with oils from the smaller fish). Whereas, a capsule the same size containing oil from anchovies and sardines, will contain, on average, 180mg of EPA and 120mg of DHA. So, we can get twice as much Omega 3 from the small fish than from the salmon, even though the capsules are the same size.

The next level of concentration involves concentrating the fish oils. The "extra strength" Omega 3 capsules will offer 400mg of EPA and 200mg of DHA per capsule, twice what the small fish provide. My concern with the higher strength products is, that when we concentrate something, we are trading off other components: including elements that may have more value than we are currently aware of. Let's look at soy foods as an example of how this process goes astray.

We start off observing dietary patterns of a culture. Japanese have lower heart disease rates and we attribute this, in part, to the ability of soy protein to lower cholesterol. Before long we have soy protein shakes and then isolated soy isoflavones in capsules. However, every time the Japanese fellow has some tofu or tempeh, he is eating it instead of meat. And he probably has some seaweed with it. The seaweed is important, since soy has a tendency to slow down thyroid function and seaweed, with it's iodine content, counteracts this tendency. This combination contributes to his overall health. By the time we have replaced a dietary component with a pill, we are far removed from the population studies that supported the health benefits of the food, in the first place.

Likewise, the Inuit had a cholesterol level that was off the charts, but, up until they started eating a modern diet, they experienced virtually no heart disease. This was due mainly to the large amounts of Omega 3 oils in their traditional diet. But again: they ate fish instead of meat. If I take a fish oil pill with my steak and fries, am I really going to get the same benefits that eating fish offers? (No.)

That being said, there is one advantage to the fish oil pill, over eating the fish, and that is that the oils (when purchased from a reputable company) will have been either processed in such a manner as to remove any mercury, or other toxic compounds, or tested for such compounds, that are often found in the flesh of the fish currently inhabiting our polluted oceans.

There is one other level of tampering that goes on, aside from concentrated fish oil products, which is based on the standard Western reductionism approach. Now that we have reduced a dietary system to a pill and concentrated that original material we take it to the next step, pharmaceutical in nature, which is to further divide the Omega 3's into separate DHA and EPA products.

Products that are almost exclusively DHA are marketed for mental acuity and those that are dominantly EPA are marketed for depression and inflammation. While some studies have indicated that isolated EPA is more effective for treating bipolar disorders and schizophrenia, generally speaking we are better off taking the whole structure of the oil. Limited studies have implied that high levels of isolate EPA may deplete the body of DHA, which makes perfect sense, since these things exist together in nature for a reason. We have seen this tendency already in the family of B vitamins and the components of vitamin E.

CHOOSING A PRODUCT

When choosing a fish oil product the first choice is between liquid and capsule. Next is the choice between a regular gelatin capsule and one that is "enteric-coated." Liquid is the best choice. A teaspoon is equal to about 4 capsules of the oil from the small fish, and is much easier to use when needing therapeutic doses to treat inflammatory conditions. In such cases one would need 8 or 12 capsules equivalent to 2 or 3 teaspoons. Most of these oils are almost tasteless when added to a protein shake. I have even put a teaspoon of high quality fish oil in my yogurt or oatmeal, and barely noticed the taste. As well, a liquid is less processed than a capsule, which requires heat in its production.

Often when people take the fish oil capsules they get it "repeating" on them. That is they burp fish-taste. This is because the capsule in not taken with a meal containing fat. When you swallow a pill, there is no signal from the mouth to the stomach as to what is coming down, and which enzymes are needed to properly digest it. Therefore, fish oils should be taken at meals where you are eating fat. The important thing is that your body knows that fat is on its way down, and this will usually improve the digestion of the oil and forbid any "repeating" of fish-taste.

For those with highly weak or sensitive digestion, there are the enteric-coated capsules that are protected against stomach acid, and they will only digest once they reach the intestinal tract. These will not "repeat" on you, even if you take them with a fat-free meal. On the other hand, their absorption will still be reduced if there is no fat at all accompanying them.

OMEGA 6

When looking at supplementing with Essential Fatty Acids, the most complicated aspect is determining how much Omega 6 Fatty Acids to utilize. Often people will pick up a 3-6-9 product, which is sold as a more balanced mix of fatty acids, and in the form of a liquid (such as "Udo's Oil" or hemp oil), this is an ideal balance of fats. That is, if you have an ideal diet.

Before we get to diet, be aware that none of these products have any appreciable level of Omega 9. That is found in Olive oil, which is one of the most healthful oils that we can consume (ideally as an Extra Virgin oil, meaning no heat or solvents were used in producing it). The now famous "Mediterranean Diet" describes the traditional dietary patterns found in the areas around Greece and Southern Italy. This diet is based on a low amount of dairy, fish and poultry in combination with low red meat intake, and low to moderate amounts of red wine.

While the Mediterranean countries consume high amounts of fat they have much less heart disease than the Western countries, much akin the phenomenon known as the "French Paradox." It is believed that the use of olive oil, as the principle source of fat in the diet, rather than meat and damaged (i.e. heated or hydrogenated) vegetable oils, is the reason for the difference in heart disease rates. Olive oil has anti-inflammatory properties and can lower cholesterol levels, blood pressure and blood sugar levels, and so deserves a prominent place in your pantry.

3-6-9 PRODUCTS

The 3-6-9 capsules are one-third fish oil, one-third flax oil and one-third borage oil. Fish and flax provide omega 3, but flax oil in a capsule is a waste of time, since it would require about 15 capsules to equal the tablespoon of flax oil required to meet your basic omega 3 requirements. The same holds true with "Udo's Oil" or hemp oil, or any vegetable oil in a capsule. A teaspoon of fish oil will be roughly equal to a tablespoon of flax oil, because it is a pre-formed Omega 3, whereas your body must convert the flax oil into Omega 3. Thus, 3 or 4 fish oil capsules would be roughly comparable to 15 flax oil capsules.

Fish oil companies will debate the conversion of flax oil into Omega 3 in their literature, but the fact is that over 700 million Hindus (a vegetarian culture/religion) managed to survive thus far, without eating any fish and without showing any major Omega 3 deficiencies (at least when following their traditional diet).

So, here's the scenario: we discover that the average North American has 10 to 20 times more Omega 6 in their diet than Omega 3. Since byproducts of Omega 6, when in excess in the body, are linked to causing inflammation, we hold this dietary imbalance responsible for contributing to diabetes, cancer, heart disease, arthritis and Alzheimer's disease, all of which are inflammatory in nature.

Realizing this, the astute student stops consuming Omega 6's (found in most commercial, restaurant and processed foods) and starts focusing on Omega 3's, using flax oil and consuming fish and fish oils. Eventually, one could end up deficient in Omega 6 fatty acids, which are still considered "essential" fatty acids, meaning the body must obtain them from an external source. For a woman this usually shows up as hormonal imbalance, such as PMS or menopausal symptoms. For a man it is trickier to know when he is deficient in Omega 6.

GLA

Omega 6 fatty acids are found in the following oils: corn, safflower, sesame, soy and sunflower. In other words, in almost all commercially used oils except canola, and canola is a dubious choice, being a hybrid (or genetically modified version) of rapeseed oil, which is toxic to humans and animals. Now, Omega 6, in its biologically active form, is known as GLA (gamma linolenic acid). While much of Omega 6 fatty acids turn into "arachidonic acid" promoting inflammation, the end product GLA may in fact reduce inflammation, in some circumstances. GLA has been used to treat auto-immune conditions, multiple sclerosis, eczema (psoriasis usually responds better to omega 3s) and PMS. One problem is that many people are unable to convert Omega 6 into GLA in their bodies, due to poor health (including alcoholism) and a lack of ancillary nutrients, which include magnesium, zinc and the vitamins C, B-3 and B-6.

GLA is found preformed in Evening Primrose Seed Oil, Borage Seed Oil, Black Current Seed Oil and Hemp Oil. Hemp oil is two-thirds Omega 6, with some GLA, and one third Omega 3, but, since it is a vegetable oil, it needs to be taken in a liquid form, as opposed to capsules (again, unless you prefer taking 15 capsules daily). The other more concentrated seed oils are often used in capsule form, with Borage being the most common in 3-6-9 formulas. While Borage is stronger in GLA, and less expensive than EPO, my preference is EPO, as a better source of effective GLA than Borage oil. And at least one study that I found showed a benefit for eczema sufferers when they took EPO, but none for those taking Borage Seed Oil.

CONFUSED?

So, what should you supplement with? Well, let's say you have a relatively standard diet. You eat in restaurants a few times a week, buy commercial salad dressings, but aren't eating wild, deep-water fish three or more times per week. You should simply take fish oil and/or flax oil, especially if you have any inflammatory conditions. If you have eczema or a hormonal imbalance, try an Evening Primrose oil product for a while (3000mg daily for therapy; 1000mg daily for maintenance).

If you have an impeccable diet (including some deep-water fish) and you avoid all processed and commercial foods, and only use olive oil at home (and coconut oil, for high heat cooking), then you are a candidate for the ideal ratio of Omega 3 to Omega 6, which would be available in Hemp or "Udo's Oil", in liquid form. Take one to two tablespoons daily on food or added to smoothies or shakes.

Most clients whom I discuss this subject with are somewhere in between the extremes. Not too many commercial foods, but not a perfect diet either. My advice to them, and to others with a similar diet, is to alternate oils on a monthly basis. One month on "Udo's Oil" or Hemp oil, the following month on flax or fish oil. This method keeps the emphasis on the Omega 3's, with enough Omega 6 to cover the bases.

Now, just to make it slightly more confusing, I will add one more thing. I do not like the taste of "Udo's Oil", although I know people who love the taste. I do not like hemp oil either, but I do like flax oil. And, I found out later that, based on the Blood Type Diet (which we will discuss in Part Two), I should not have "Udo's Oil", because it contains sunflower and sesame seed oils, which do not agree with my blood type. The point here is that, when dealing with real foods (as opposed to junk foods and processed foods), we can listen to feedback from our taste buds. I stick with fish and flax oils, and if I feel the need to have some Omega 6, I will pick up some reputable Evening Primrose oil capsules.

Finally, remember that bad fats steal good fats. That is, damaged oils (over-heated and hydrogenated vegetable oils) and excessive saturated fats, will rob the body of good fatty acids. When the body wants Essential Fatty Acids it will crave fat indiscriminately. You may be craving potato chips and deep fried foods when what your body really needs is Omega 3, 6 and/or 9.

CLOSING

Now that you have most of your nutritional bases covered, you will be taking up to 5 or more pills per day. For the sake of convenience, a variety of pre-made multi-packs are available. These packs include from 3 to 9 pills per serving. In the case of the larger pill packs you will find most of what was discussed above, as well as extras. Some also provide "super- foods" such as kelp and alfalfa, for their iodine and other trace minerals, "greens" for their detoxifying and alkalizing effects, and adrenal-supportive herbs, like Siberian Ginseng, for fighting stress and supporting energy levels. Better products will offer digestive enzymes to improve the absorption of the nutrients and the meal that they are taken with. Look also for bonus antioxidants such as Alpha Lipoic Acid, Grape Seed Extract and Quercetin, that complement and enhance the basic nutritional antioxidants (A, C, E and Selenium).

Remember, almost all vitamins, minerals and fatty acids need to be taken with food. As I mentioned with EFA's, fat-soluble nutrients (A, D, E, K, Fatty Acids, COQ10, Alpha Lipoic Acid, etc) especially benefit from being taken at a meal that contains some fat in it. Often overlooked is the premise that digestion begins in the mouth. When we swallow a pill containing fat-soluble nutrients, without chewing fat, the stomach has no signal that it should release "Lipase," the fat-digesting enzyme. Therefore generally consume supplements that contain these nutrients at a meal that contains some fat (this includes meat, fish, eggs, poultry, tofu, salad dressing) for optimal assimilation.

When choosing a supplement we must also appreciate that Timed Release is considered a passé technology, as it was discovered (some time ago) that B-vitamins are absorbed up in the upper intestinal tract, whereas pills inevitably sink to the lower intestinal tract. Timed release has also been considered of dubious value when applied to regular vitamin C. Since, as I've mentioned, ascorbic acid is so acidic that chewable (non-buffered) vitamin C is worse on the teeth than sugar, it has been suggested (in "Life Extension"; Durk Pearson and Sandy Shaw; 1983; Warner Books, NY, New York) that this pill will ultimately sink to the lower intestinal tract, and there drip acid for 8 hrs, potentially ulcerating the lining of the gut.

Now, a brief word about swallowing a large number of pills at mealtime. Washing pills down with a cup of liquid has the side effect of diluting the stomach acid, which reduces the digestibility of everything. Try swallowing the pills with the food, as you eat. One does not need to chew the pill, just slip it into the mouth prior to swallowing the masticated food. An added benefit of this technique is, that the throat opens wider for food than liquid, so for those with difficulty swallowing, even large pills go down easily.

Please, be aware that each of the supplements addressed here is worthy of a book of its' own. And most of them already have more than one book written about their many values. My overview has indeed been as a "generalist" and if I have missed an important attribute of one of your favorite nutrients, forgive me. Such an approach necessitates that we cannot cover everything. Don't let that stop you from exploring on your own. If a particular nutrient hits a note with you, dig deeper: This subject matter is endlessly fascinating and the payoff is well worth the effort, since it will contribute to you, and your loved ones', health and happiness.

PART TWO:

SUPPLEMENTS FOR GENERAL HEALTH AND WELL BEING

CHAPTER ONE

PROTECT YOUR BRAIN WITH VITAMIN B12

As mentioned in part one, I am devoting a separate chapter to the benefits of vitamin B-12, specifically because many of you are aging "boomers." There is no more affordable way to prevent mental deterioration during aging, than ensuring a more than adequate supply of vitamin B-12.

WHAT IS B-12?

Vitamin B-12, or cobalamin, is a red crystalline substance isolated in 1948, when it was determined to prevent pernicious anemia, a red blood cell deficiency. Later, it was discovered to be important in energy, immune and nerve functions. Whereas the other B vitamins are water-soluble, B-12 is stored in the body, especially in the kidneys and liver. It can take years of inadequate intake, or declining digestive ability, before a severe deficiency shows up. Unfortunately, when a severe deficiency does show up, it manifests as damage to the brain and nervous system, which may occur without ever first revealing itself as anemia.

WHY DO WE NEED TO SUPPLEMENT WITH B-12?

Our stomachs normally secrete a digestive compound called "intrinsic factor", that helps the body to absorb vitamin B-12 through the small intestine. Certain conditions cause "intrinsic factor" to decline, including reduced stomach acid, which occurs in certain blood types (type A and AB) and/or with aging and a strict vegetarian diet. It has been estimated that at least 10% to 30% of those 50 and older have decreased stomach acid secretion, to the point of impeding the absorption of B-12 from food. Also, those with conditions that inflame or irritate the stomach (including Crohn's disease and colitis) may stop producing intrinsic factor, a double negative since the B-12 would help to heal the lining of the stomach and intestines.

Vitamin B-12 is only readily available in the diet from animal protein. The highest amounts being found in kidney, liver, meat, eggs, fish and cheese. While it appears to exist in fermented soy products, such as tempeh and miso, and in algae such as spirulina, most experts agree that this is an analogue form. That is, it looks like B-12 under a microscope, but doesn't actually function as such in the body. In fact, analogues are believed by some to occupy the receptors in the body and forbid the proper uptake of the real nutrient. As mentioned in Part One, this certainly occurs with the analogue of vitamin E, where the synthetic version (from petroleum) blocks the uptake of natural vitamin E.

I like to point out to "Vegans" (those who eat no animal based products) that there is no historical precedent for veganism amongst humans. No culture in history has ever totally avoided animal foods. Traditionally, the Hindus (a vegetarian religion/culture) eat no meat, fish or eggs, but consume dairy foods, while the Japanese eat no dairy, but consume fish and eggs and, like the Chinese, also consume small amounts of meat (again, we are talking about traditional diets).

To my knowledge the only recorded vegan group is a religious sect of East Indians called "Jains", whose non-violent path eliminates all animal foods; to the degree that they go to great lengths to avoid killing insects, or even bacteria. No one has analyzed their diet for B-12 deficiency, but the indicators are good that it is prevalent among them, as it has been found to be extremely common in even strict vegetarians.

Media reports recently told the tale of a serious B-12 deficiency found in the offspring of vegan parents, to the point where their child was in danger of dying. Unfortunately, in the past four years there have been 3 manslaughter convictions against vegan parents for the deaths of their infants, in the United States (www.naturalhygienesociety.org). In one case they fed their infant only soy milk and fruit juice, until the child's death at 6 weeks. It was pointed out, in reports on this case, that even the breast milk of a strict vegan mother will be dangerously lacking in the Omega 3 fatty acid DHA, which is required for eye and brain development in infants.

SUBLINGUAL B12

Because of this tendency towards mal-absorption, the medical profession uses injection to provide patients with a guaranteed amount of B-12. Another way to bypass the need for "intrinsic factor" is to take the supplement under the tongue, which allows it to enter the blood stream through the mucous membranes. Less uncomfortable than an injection and just as effective, this simple method can be used without the need to see a doctor. Sublingual B-12 is available in little lozenges made of lactose or sorbitol, or in a glycerin-based, liquid form.

METHYLCOBALAMIN

The last generation of vitamin B-12 in supplemental form was known as "cyanocobalamin," as cyanide was involved in the process of synthesizing it. This was an inactive form and required conversion by the liver into something that could be utilized. The newest form is known as "methylcobalamin," and is considered an active form of the vitamin, immediately available for use by the body. This is the form of B-12 found to be most active in the central nervous system. In fact, studies comparing cyanocobalamin to methylcobalamin, in cancerous rats, showed that only the methyl form prolonged their lifespan.

THE MANY FUNCTIONS OF B-12

Most importantly, vitamin B-12 (along with folic acid) is required to synthesize DNA, build red blood cells, and to maintain the myelin sheath that holds nerve cells together and conducts signals along the nerves. This makes it critical to prevent neurological diseases, including Multiple Sclerosis, Parkinson's disease and ALS. It has been estimated by some researchers that if doctors were liberal with B-12 injections, they could cut senile dementia rates amongst seniors in half. Deficiency of B-12 is also linked to depression and Alzheimer's disease in the elderly.

A recent study involving 100 seniors, confirmed that those with inadequate levels of B-12 are more prone to brain atrophy (Neurology 2008: 71). These participants, ranging from 60 to 90 years old, were examined yearly using cognitive tests, MRI scans and blood tests. Over years, it was found that the individuals with the least amount of B-12 in their bodies had six times the brain shrinkage of those with the highest amounts. The critical thing to observe in this study is that none of the participants would have actually met the medical criteria for B-12 deficiency. They all registered within the low-normal range. This is because blood levels of B-12 (which is the indicator measured) do not accurately reflect what the tissue levels are.

In one limited study, involving 39 seniors, patients were treated for neurological problems with B-12 injections. All showed some degree of improvement, ranging from slight to dramatic, in symptoms of abnormal gait, poor reflexes, memory loss, muscle weakness, fatigue and psychiatric problems. As well, supplementing with B-12 has clearly shown that it improves cognition, especially the ability to recall words.

Vitamin B-12 is also required for the cells with a high turnover rate, including those that line the internal mucosal membrane, from the top orifice to the bottom one. (Which makes it a co-worker with the aforementioned vitamins A and D.) This function of forming and maintaining cells makes it essential for the health of the reproductive organs and the lungs. The value of B-12 for the lungs was well demonstrated in an experiment that studied 73 long-time, heavy smokers. It has been known for some time that cigarette smoke lowers the levels of B-12 and folic acid in the cells of the lungs and bronchioles. The smokers were divided into two groups, one group getting supplemental B-12 along with folic acid and the other getting a placebo. Within four months of treatment the group that got the vitamins showed far fewer pre-cancerous cells than the control group.

Other functions that are dependent on adequate levels of B-12 include digestion, nutrient absorption and the metabolism of fats and carbohydrates. Some doctors have even successfully used B-12 injections to help speed recovery from surgery, as well as from bacterial and viral infections. As discussed in Part One, along with vitamin B-6 and folic acid, vitamin B-12 helps to keep homocysteine levels in check. (High homocysteine allows cholesterol to trap in the arteries, leading to atherosclerosis.)

METHYLATION AND MOOD

Vitamin B-12 is also involved in the process of methylation, via a regeneration of the amino acid methionine and a synthesis of SamE. The biochemical process of methylation in the body requires SamE (S-adenosylmethionine, pronounced "sammy") for virtually all of its functions. We know now that free radicals do the majority of their damage by inhibiting methylation. By maintaining and enhancing methylation in the body we are actively fighting premature aging, as well as cancer and heart disease.

SamE is needed for over a hundred enzymatic reactions in the body, including those for reduction of inflammation, liver health and mood regulation. Dementia symptoms caused by B-12 deficiency look very much like Alzheimer's disease, and Alzheimer's disease is often accompanied by a deficiency of both B-12 and SamE. Vitamin B-12 and SamE produce and promote the activity of the neurotransmitters dopamine and serotonin, necessary for a healthy emotional state, and the hormone melatonin, required for a proper sleep cycle.

As an illustration of the importance of B-12 on emotional states, we look to a study done on 122 severely depressed women. The subjects with the worst B-12 deficiency (27%) were over twice as likely to be severely depressed as the non-deficient women. Another hospital review found that up to 30% of patients hospitalized for depression, were deficient in B-12.

DEFICIENCY SYMPTOMS

- Nerve damage due to B-12 deficiency shows up first as an aggressive tingling sensation, or a burning or numbing sensation in the extremities.
- Neurological damage and headaches: Maintains the fatty sheaths that protect nerve endings.
- Due to its support of the mucosal membranes, deficiency can show up as a red, swollen tongue and/or consistent diarrhea.
- Asthma, including childhood asthma.
- Diabetic Neuropathy.
- Reduced fertility: B-12 can improve sperm count and motility.
- Tinnitus: Ringing in the ear, as well as noise-induced hearing loss.
- Sleep disorders: B-12 helps to make Melatonin in the body.
- Depression: B-12 is involved in the activity of dopamine.
- Anxiety: B-12 is involved in the activity of serotonin.

- Extreme fatigue and poor appetite.
- Sulfite sensitivity. Subjects allergic to sulfites were given 2,000mcg of B-12 before exposure to the offending substance, and all but one avoided all allergic reactions (congestion, headache, runny nose and bronchial spasms).

DRUGS THAT INTERFERE WITH B-12 ABSORPTION

Antibiotics; Anticoagulant drugs; Anticonvulsants; Gout medications; Blood pressure medications; Birth control pills; Cholesterol lowering drugs; Parkinson's medications.

While not a drug, one should be aware that high levels of folic acid, in supplemental form, can mask a B-12 deficiency. This is why, in Canada, folic acid is limited to 1 mg in any daily supplement. Folic acid will correct a deficiency in blood cells but will not correct B12 deficiency in the brain, resulting in brain damage if B-12 deficiency is treated with folic acid for too long. In fact, excessive folic acid, in the absence of sufficient B-12, can worsen neurological problems. Deficiency in either folic acid or B-12 will accelerate a deficiency in the other. So when supplementing with one, ensure that you get a supplemental amount of the other. Usually, obtaining at least 1mg of folic acid, at least 5 days per week, should be sufficient.

DOSAGE

Most supplements provide 1,000 mcg (1mg) of B-12 per serving. If you are deficient in B-12 it is suggested that one takes 2,000mcg daily for one month, followed by 1,000mcg daily thereafter for another month. A blood test can be done to see if severe deficiency has been rectified. Dosages for infertility run as high as 6,000mcg daily, while for neurological conditions, such as Multiple Sclerosis and Parkinson's disease, they may go as high as 60,000mcg daily (60mg).

Since we cannot count on a medical test to definitively indicate if we need more B-12 (much like the current vitamin D test, and thyroid test), it would serve us well to be proactive with this vitamin. For those nearing 50 and older, who suspect a need for B-12, I usually suggest that they take 5000mcg daily for 5 days, and see if they feel differently. Usually this manifests as a reduction in "brain fog" and an increase in physical energy. If nothing is noticeable, or when noticeable benefits cease, a small amount can be used for maintaining brain protection. This amounts to about 1,000mcg five days a week, or 5,000mcg once per week (in sublingual form).

While no toxicity has ever been recorded with regards to B-12, as usual I suggest that you do not take it 7 days a week. At the very least, skip weekends and reduce dosage when you feel your deficiency has been eliminated. While it may be very safe, we still do not wish to create a dependency on the supplement, except in extreme cases where the B-12 is serving a pharmaceutical, therapeutic function.

CHAPTER TWO

THIS IS A PROTEIN: THIS IS A CARB

You may think you know all about protein and carbohydrates and, if so, you can consider this a refresher course. If you don't know that much about them, then this will serve as a fitness and sports-primer on the proper use of protein and carbs, for building and/or maintaining lean muscle tissue, while burning unwanted body fat.

The origins of this chapter began as an article for the early "Cops for Cancer Run". It was just a basic run down of how to properly use protein shakes (which were relatively new to the market then) and carbohydrates for exercise, endurance and burning excess body fat. My idea of an amusing title was (in its' full form) "This is a protein, this is a carb, this one's for muscle and this one's for lard." This brilliant take-off on the military ditty ("This is my rifle this is my gun...") went nowhere, since no one "got it" (except for our contact with the police department).

Nonetheless, to this day I find many people still don't know the basics. I have had people ask me if there is enough protein in a carrot (no), and even athletes (including one who went on to the Olympics) were ignorant of these basics, even though they had professional coaches. So, you might be surprised at what you don't know about protein and carbs.

WHAT IS PROTEIN?

Protein is made up of chains of amino acids, and conventional food sources include meat, fish, poultry, eggs and dairy products. Beans and legumes are also moderately high in protein, with soybeans being the richest of these. While seeds and nuts do contain a moderately high amount of protein, it is usually difficult to eat enough of them to meet high protein requirements.

Protein is the building block for muscle, glands, hair, ligaments, nails, tendons, and organs. It is required for growing, healing and repairing bones, cells and tissues. The amino acids are also required for neurotransmitter production, and so, affect mood and mental states. In other words, protein is of critical importance to the body and its health.

In the absence of sufficient protein, physical exertion whether aerobic, weight training, or just a vigorous walk, will cause the body to consume muscle instead of fat. This is because exercise causes stress and damage to the muscles that have been worked. These muscles then require amino acids, particularly L-glutamine and the branch chain amino acids, to repair themselves.

If a reserve of amino acids, from recently consumed protein, is not available for immediate use, the body will then pirate it from its own undamaged muscle tissue. One has about 30 to 45 minutes after exertion to ingest a high quality protein, in order to ensure that fat will be burned, instead of muscle. Protein itself will not convert to fat, however, when it is found in animal products, protein is usually accompanied by saturated fat, which can be fattening when consumed in excess.

Since meat can require more than an hour to be properly digested, a pre-digested protein powder shake becomes the obvious choice for supporting tissue repair, and reducing fatigue and recovery time.

Protein from soy sources, including tofu, tempeh and soymilk, can help the body to burn fat by accelerating the metabolism. This only applies, however, if one ingests reasonable amounts of iodine in the diet (from seaweed or as a supplement), otherwise soy foods can slow down thyroid function, having the opposite effect. Soy products can also help to balance female hormones and reduce cholesterol, however soy is a common allergen, and therefore not suitable for everyone. Because there is a lot of controversy about soy foods these days, I will address the subject in more detail towards the end of this chapter.

PROTEIN POWDERS

As a supplement, powdered protein is available in the forms of egg, hemp, pea, pumpkin, rice, soy and whey. (I will be referring to whey from cow's milk, but there is also goat milk protein and whey on the market. Although there is not much science on goat whey, it is rich in minerals and useful for digestive disorders, and easier to digest than cow whey, for some people.) Some professionals suggest that proteins should be rotated, to avoid habituation to the effects of always using the same amino acid profile (each different protein will have a different mix of dominant amino acids). So, if we use whey protein for one month, we might choose a vegetable protein for the following month. But of all the proteins available, whey is the preferred choice in the sports kingdom.

This is because it is the only protein that will enhance immune function, by raising glutathione levels in the body. Endurance athletes especially, are prone to lung infections because they push their bodies so hard. After it was found that those on whey protein had less infections and better recovery times, it became the dominant protein used by most athletes. This is also why whey is the best choice for feeding those who are very ill or recovering from illness. Or those coping with muscular-wasting diseases, since whey is also very high (24%) in the "Branch Chain Amino Acids", which are three amino acids specific to maintaining and building muscle mass.

Even though whey is derived from milk, those who are lactose-intolerant can use a whey protein "isolate", which will have virtually no lactose in it. Whey isolates also have next to no fat in them; for those worried about antibiotic or growth hormone residues in the whey, as a result of modern dairy practices, rest assured that all such residues reside in the fat. The cheaper whey "concentrates," will contain some lactose and fat. An isolate is about 80 to 90% protein, whereas a whey concentrate is generally about 68% protein, and will contain 5 to 8% lactose (and is considerably cheaper to purchase). In order to determine the actual amount of protein in a product that you are considering purchasing, simply divide the amount of protein per serving by the serving size. Therefore, if there is 24grams of protein per serving and the serving size is 30grams, we divide 24 by 30 to get the number .8, which equals 80% protein.

HOW MUCH PROTEIN?

In order to attain muscle growth or to encourage fat loss, via exercise, one must ingest quality protein from 4 to 6 times per day. The servings should be evenly divided throughout the day, from morning to evening, at roughly 2 to 3 hours apart. Servings of protein should not generally exceed 30 grams per meal, and the most critical times to consume protein are first thing in the morning and after exercise. It is not necessary (but is acceptable) to have protein before exercise, but if you skip breakfast consider having a protein shake in the morning. This is because by middle age we tend to muscular waste if we do not have protein in the morning, having essentially "fasted" for the previous eight hours.

Our daily protein requirements range from approximately half a gram of protein per pound of body weight, for a sedentary lifestyle, to a full gram of protein per pound of bodyweight, for a vigorous muscle building or weight loss program. Such a program, involving high levels of protein, is usually only advised for a duration of three to six months, before returning to a more moderate intake.

So, if you weighed 120 lbs and did little by the way of physical activity, you would require about 60 grams of protein per day (in divided doses, since most of us can not utilize more than 30 grams in a sitting, and even that amount is usually only required after physical exertion). Also, if you were trying to reshape your body, you would require about 120 grams of protein per day. In this case, along with ensuring that one has some protein at each of the three daily meals, an additional 2 or 3 servings of protein per day, between the main meals, should suffice.

At this point you may want to obtain a protein chart, which will give you an idea of the protein content of most foods. Prepackaged foods and protein powders will list their protein content on the label, but it is a good idea to get an overview on the protein content of the foods you commonly eat. Such charts are available in book form, on-line or often as a handout in health food and supplement stores.

CARBOHYDRATES

No matter what Dr. Atkins said, not all carbs are evil. (He created "The Atkins' Diet," which advocated a high protein and fat diet, along with extreme carbohydrate restriction, for weight loss purposes.) He was (he is now deceased) correct about refined (or "simple") carbohydrates (those with the fiber removed), which function like sugars in the body, raising blood sugar levels and thus insulin levels. Of course, the carbohydrates commonly found in the standard North American diet are mostly refined (e.g. fruit juice, sodas, sugar, white rice, white potatoes, breads and pasta) and do contribute to both fat storage and diabetes. But, complex carbohydrates, such as whole grains and yams, are not fattening, due to their high fiber content, which slows insulin release.

When insulin is high, the body will store carbs as fat. This does not occur however, in that 45-minute window of opportunity after physical exertion. During this time, carbs, no matter how refined, will replenish glycogen stores in the liver and muscles, providing fuel for the following day's exertions. This is what is known as "carb-loading" and only occurs after exercise. What is often over-looked by amateur athletes is that one cannot carb-load before exercise.

THE TRUTH ABOUT CARB-LOADING

Carbohydrates ingested before exercise will be used as fuel by the body, instead of stored body fat. Refined carbs, for someone trying to lose body fat, are only of value after exertion is well under way (in a diluted liquid form, for endurance events), and after exercise is over. I describe the process to people in evolutionary terms: We ran it down, killed it and ate it, absorbing nutrients in order to run it down again, tomorrow. It might be hunting (protein and fat) or gathering (carbohydrates mainly), but the exertion is followed by nutrient absorption, facilitating the process for the following days.

This principle is missing from the "Atkins" approach to weight loss. Instead of totally denying carbohydrates to his adherents, ensuring that no one could maintain the diet for any length of time, he could have offered the "carrot and stick" approach. If you take the "stick," exercise, you get the "carrot" (carrot cake if you desire), since these carbs are not fattening, after exercise. We do need a certain amount of carbohydrates in the diet, since they are involved in producing serotonin, our calming neurotransmitter necessary for relaxing and sleeping.

After exercise, one should accompany the 30 or so grams of protein (20-25gr for women) with 60 to 90 grams of carbohydrates (depending on exercise intensity). If you cannot get the carbs from a meal, soon enough after completing your exercise (from potatoes, pasta, rice, etc.), then a glass of orange juice (or most fruit juice) has about 30 grams of carbs, and a banana about the same.

So, blending these in with your protein will pretty much cover that requirement.

Remember that the 30 grams of carbs in a glass of orange juice is roughly equal to a glass of soda pop, and aside from a little added synthetic vitamin C, it is about as healthy for you as a glass of pop. Especially from the perspective of weight-loss, since those on a weight loss program generally need to reduce their overall carb intake and increase their protein intake.

Many people are unaware that carbohydrates are the most fattening substance that we eat: more so than even fat. In fact, a low fat diet will only convince the body that there is a famine, and it will conserve body fat, making it even more difficult to burn it off. This is especially true for women, since nature wishes to ensure that they have enough body fat storage to get them through a pregnancy and nursing, should famine occur.

PROTEIN SHAKES

High quality protein isolates are theoretically best taken in water, but a small trade off in absorption is usually worth the increase in taste value to be gained by mixing it into juice (post-workout), or a milk-like substance (almond, hemp, rice or soy). Cow milk is generally not advisable for those on weight loss programs. Remember that the milk from a cow is a biological program to build the body of a cow. (Whey is a fraction of the cow's milk, and leaves behind the milk protein, casein, or "curds," which is the more allergenic component of milk.) Yogurt, because it is fermented, is easier to digest, and a more suitable dairy product. Even better for humans is goat milk, which is closer in mineral and lactose composition to human milk.

Because pure protein powders are usually made without carbohydrates, they are commonly sweetened with artificial sweeteners (or left unsweetened). I suggest you research any artificial sweetener before including it as a regular part of your diet. Currently, sucralose is considered to be the safest artificial sweetener. Still I would not give it to children, since ten years down-line we usually find out that the latest artificial sweetener wasn't as safe as we were led to believe.

"Stevia" is a viable alternative to artificial sweeteners. Stevia is safe, natural, does not raise blood sugar levels, and does not feed candida yeast in the body like regular sugars do. Stevia has been used for decades as a safe sweetener for diabetics, in Brazil and Japan. It has been illegal to use as a sweetener in North America due to the lobbying influence on the governmental bodies by the manufacturers of artificial sweeteners. That is now changing due to Coke and Pepsi applying for the rights to use Stevia in soft drinks.

A protein shake makes a great evening snack, but should be taken without any appreciable level of carbohydrates. Ingesting simple carbs within 2 to 3 hours of going to sleep will cause your growth hormone levels to drop, due to the insulin spike they cause. Since growth hormone allows us to burn fat and build muscle while we sleep, it helps us to maintain a youthful muscle-to-fat ratio.

ADDING GOOD FATS

Contrary to the low-fat diet concept, we find that by giving the body good fats (i.e. Essential Fatty Acids), such as flax seed oil, extra virgin olive oil, or fish, we can convince it to use stored fat as a fuel. Currently popular for this purpose is the use of extra virgin coconut oil, which appears to hasten fat burning more than most oils. This may be because it stimulates the thyroid gland to increase ones' metabolism. Because coconut oil is hard at room temperature, it won't be ideal for adding to your shake.

It is now common for those using a protein shake (with or without carbs) to add a tablespoon of nutritive oils (flax, hemp, Udo's, etc; or a teaspoon of fish oil) to each shake. This slows the transit time of the protein through the digestive system, allowing for better assimilation. Since the protein powders are essentially pre-digested, they tend to move through the digestive tract too fast (in contrast to meat, which is too slow for post-workout purposes). By slowing down their passage, we will ensure the bio-availability of the amino acids for a longer period of time. This will enhance muscle repair and rebuilding, and just simply help you feel satisfied for longer, if you are counting on the shake to serve as a meal replacement.

Fat (as well as protein) also slows the insulin release caused by simple carbohydrates, making them less fattening. For this reason, for example, a potato with butter is likely to be less fattening than one without some fat added. Likewise, adding peanut butter to bread, or protein and olive oil to pasta, will reduce the insulin-spiking tendency of these simple carbohydrates.

CREATINE

We will now take a brief look at creatine, the single most effective sports supplement since steroids, with the advantage of being both considerably safer, and legal. But creatine is not just for extreme athletes. Because it produces ATP (adenosine triphosphate, which is, essentially, cellular energy) in the body, it is used to treat fibromyalgia, chronic fatigue syndrome, and as a follow up to heart surgery. In fact cardiologists know that having a good storage of creatine in the body can prevent brain damage from occurring during and after a stroke.

There has been some debate about the safety of creatine, but none of it is based on science. Scientifically, creatine has been proven to be both safe and effective, especially if you purchase a high quality pharmaceutical grade (usually German or Japanese) and avoid the cheap products (usually Chinese). Look for the "Creapure" logo for assured quality (German pharmaceutical grade.) There are now fancy new types of creatine available, but at this point I suggest you stick with creatine "monohydrate," the original form with the most research behind it.

Creatine is a natural substance found in meat (damaged by cooking), and produced in the body. It will make one stronger, allowing for a better workout, which in the presence of adequate protein, will build muscle faster, in turn burning fat more effectively. Women should rest assured that creatine and protein will not make you look like a man; only steroids can do that.

WOMEN AND EXERCISE

Speaking of women and exercise, many women find that their exercise is not paying off they way they would expect. This is usually because they are not ingesting the required protein and carbs within the 45-minute window of opportunity, following exercise. They are therefore burning muscle and retaining fat, and not attaining their objective. Building muscle is necessary for continual fat burning, and more important than aerobic exercise for this purpose. But, to re-emphasize, it will not create a masculine-looking body in a female, unless one focuses excessively on heavy weight training, and severely over-exercises.

Excessive exercising, along with heavy weight training, eventually causes a woman's testosterone levels to rise to the point that she will shift to a more masculine shape. By this time, she will also have ceased menstruating, indicating that this hormonal shift has occurred. I found it somewhat ironic to discuss natural breast-enhancement, with a woman who was so phobic about her body fat, that she exercised to this sort of ridiculous level. Having bought into the media image of a female with the body of a girl and the breasts of a woman, she seemed unaware that breasts are composed mostly of fat. The only way to have that cake, and eat it too, is breast-enhancement surgery.

HOW TO USE CREATINE

Now, let's get back to creatine. Creatine is usually taken three to five times daily, for five days, which is known as the "loading phase".

This gives a jump-start to the beneficial effects, but at five times per day can cause considerable water retention, so I suggest no more than three times daily, for most people. Because of this tendency towards water retention, it is important to drink extra water when using creatine, as it pulls water out of the blood. If you skip the loading phase, it will take a few weeks before the extra strength benefits become apparent.

Creatine is commonly used with 35 grams of dextrose (glucose), which is why it is taken after exercise, when the dextrose becomes part of ones' carb-load (remember to count the 35 grams as part of your 60 to 90 gram carb-load). So, a post-workout serving of creatine is one teaspoon (5 grams) with 7 teaspoons of dextrose (35 grams). This high carbohydrate intake is designed to spike the insulin levels, which then shuttles the creatine to the cells in a timely manner.

Obviously one doesn't really want that much dextrose three times per day (during the loading phase,) especially if we are trying to avoid refined sugars (and dextrose is at the top of the chart on the glycemic index). So, you can either use only 3 teaspoons of dextrose (15 grams) to one of creatine, during the "non-post-workout" times of the day, or use grape juice (which may also be used for post-workout, if you wish to avoid the dextrose). It is acceptable to add the creatine to your protein shake, but you must not add it to orange juice or coffee, as it is widely believed that these damage the creatine, and reduce or eliminate its effectiveness.

Creatine is taken once or twice daily, after the loading phase, even on non-workout days (again, don't use the full dose of dextrose on these days), for about 30 days. It is then advisable to stop using the creatine for 2 to 4 weeks, in order to ensure that the body does not shut down its own production of creatine (we produce an average of about 2 grams daily). After this period, you can begin the cycle over again, if you wish.

One alternative to spiking insulin levels with dextrose is to use a ½ teaspoon of baking soda with a full teaspoon of creatine. This effervescent reaction also improves uptake by the body. One authority has also suggested that it is more effective to simply divide the teaspoon of creatine into the three meals of the day, just sprinkling it onto the food. Both these alternatives are also recommended for anyone who finds creatine to be difficult to digest (occasionally it can cause stomach upset in some people).

L-GLUTAMINE

The isolated amino acid L-Glutamine is the third most commonly used sports and fitness supplement, with protein, of course, being number one, and creatine being number two.

Added to your protein shake, L-glutamine will improve recovery time after extreme exercise and, used during the day, will help to stabilize blood sugar levels. L-glutamine also converts to glutathione (enhancing immune and detoxification pathways), glucosamine (repairing cartilage), n-acetyl-glucosamine (for healing the lining of the intestinal tract), and works to improve mood and mental function. On top of all that, glutamine can also raise growth hormone levels.

To raise growth hormone levels (for those middle-aged and older) simply mix half a teaspoon (2 grams or more) of L-glutamine with ¼ teaspoon of baking soda, and water. Taking this mixture on an empty stomach, first thing in the morning and/or before bed, has been shown in studies to raise growth hormone levels by up to 400%. This, to a degree, rolls back the biological clock, enhancing fat burning, tissue repair and immune function.

IS SOY DANGEROUS?

It's time now for that closer look at soy protein. There is a lot of controversy surrounding the consumption of soy food products and, unfortunately in these days of purchased science, one-sided arguments, disinformation and propaganda passing for objective information, it is hard to determine what the truth is. While soy marketing information offers only the positive aspects, the other side (perhaps motivated by the dairy industry?) offers only the negative material. As usual, the truth lies in between the two extremes.

The launch of the hyper-critical material on soy products occurred under the title "Tragedy and Hype" in "Nexus" magazine, a periodical notorious for its "way out in left field" approach to its subject matter (which includes a lot of conspiratorial material). A response was issued sometime later by the "Townsend Letter for Doctors and Patients" (www.tldp.com), a somewhat more respected source (though still of an unorthodox bent).

The articles critical of soy foods tend to refer to a lot of rat and bird studies, extrapolating them to humans. Remember that rats don't have "Thalidomide babies" (which was why that drug was given to pregnant women), so they are not a great substitute for humans, in clinical trials.

Let's look at one of the main arguments that articles critical of soy postulate; the high phytic acid found in soy foods, which is a component that inhibits mineral absorption. The traditional use of soy in Oriental cultures balances its mineral-depleting tendencies by fermenting it (miso, tamari and tempeh), to neutralize the phytic acid. As well, when they consume non-fermented soy foods, such as tofu, they eat it with seafood or small amounts of meats. The extra minerals found in animal protein balances out the tendency of soy foods to inhibit some mineral absorption. Also, a diet high in meat can provide an excess of minerals to the body (especially iron and sodium), which eating some soy food can help to keep in check.

Now, the interesting thing here is, that there is an anti-cancer product on the market called IP6, a well-researched substance that is derived from phytic acid. So, if we are looking only at one property of a substance, and only one aspect of that property, we are not going to get a complete picture.

YIN AND YANG

In Western medicine, soy is considered "estrogenic" (raises the female hormone, estrogen) whereas to the Oriental system it is considered "yin," or "cooling," in nature. Animal protein (meat, especially) by contrast, is known in the West to raise testosterone (male hormone) levels, and in the East is determined to be "yang," or "heating," in nature.

We can see that soy is a good balance to a meat-based diet. Not only does it counter-act the tendency of meat to raise testosterone and over-heat the body system, but it can also reduce cholesterol levels (this is well established, scientifically), another side effect of high animal protein intake.

So, if one has high blood pressure, or hot flashes due to menopause, both of which are "heated" conditions, soy is an appropriate way to help cool the body system. If you were pale, weak and cold most of the time, your condition, already too cool, would be worsened by soy foods (and "cooling" herbs such as North American Ginseng) but improved by more "heating" foods (and herbs, such as Korean Red Ginseng).

Thus, while soy may aggravate PMS due to its estrogenic nature (most PMS is due to excessive estrogen levels), it could aid menopausal symptoms, a condition caused by low estrogen. "In good studies, soy reduces the frequency of hot flashes 20 to 30% more than a placebo does," reports M. Kurzer, the director of the Healthy Foods, Healthy Lives Institute (University of Minnesota).

The fermentation of soy foods will eliminate the estrogenic properties, so, again, miso, tamari, and tempeh, do not carry any of these concerns. I have, however, observed that the new generation of fermented soy protein isolates appears to be even more estrogenic than unfermented soy foods, and should be used only to raise estrogen levels.

The real danger of excess soy consumption occurs mostly amongst vegans, and those who use it as their only real source of protein. To have the majority of ones' protein derived from a "cooling" source would, over time, create an imbalance in the body. Traditionally all cultures that consume soy foods also consume some animal protein. On the other hand, a diet based dominantly on animal protein would also create an imbalance by being too heating. That is unless you lived in the Arctic, which being very cold requires many thermal units of energy and heat (calories), in order to survive. Vegetarian cultures tend towards existing in hot climates, since they can get away with less calories (and "heat").

Other arguments against the use of soy include the fact that soybeans contain enzyme inhibitors. These are also found in any raw seed or nut (the reason Eastern systems advise against consuming them raw) and are neutralized by simply cooking, fermenting or sprouting the food (or even just soaking in water for 24 hours, in the case of seeds and nuts).

It is true that soy foods dampen thyroid function and, considering the vast majority of Westerners have poorly functioning thyroids, it is important that people are aware of this. Again, traditionally, any culture that consumes soy foods also consumes seaweed, so it is important if you use soy foods regularly, that you also ensure an adequate iodine intake.

This means eating seaweed regularly, or at least obtaining the Recommended Daily Allowance of iodine (150mcg) through nutritional supplementation. While this amount is too low for optimal thyroid health (the Japanese get 20 times this much; a subject to be addressed in my next book), it should be sufficient to offset the thyroid-inhibiting tendencies of soy foods.

WHAT TO LOOK FOR WHEN BUYING SOY

Certainly there are arguments to be made against consuming soy products that are non-organic, particularly since almost all non-organic soybeans are genetically modified. And this particular modification allows the plant to take more of the pesticide "Round-up," than the last generation of soybean. Surprisingly, the company that genetically modifies the soybean also manufactures "Round-up," which sounds like a win-win proposition: for someone.

Aside from ensuring that our soy foods are organic, there is another thing to be aware of, with regards to tofu. A friend who worked in a tofu plant informed me that there is a distinction in quality between the tofu that uses calcium sulfate as a coagulant and those that use magnesium chloride. The calcium sulfate (which is a cheaper ingredient) in the tofu is believed to impede mineral digestion, while the magnesium chloride encourages it.

This information made me recall the Hawaiian study, that linked tofu consumption to Alzheimer's disease among immigrant Japanese. Recently, it has come to my attention that soybeans will pick up aluminum, if it is in the soil, and we know that high aluminum levels in the brain are linked to Alzheimer's disease. It turns out that both magnesium and aluminum compete for the same receptor sites in the body, therefore, it is plausible that using magnesium chloride in the tofu, may forbid the body from up-taking any aluminum that may be found in the product.

Contrary to claims made in the Nexus article, and others of its persuasion, there are no studies on humans that show negative effects of soy foods on offspring. I personally raised three healthy boys to adulthood on a relatively high soy diet, and their mother consumed a lot of soy foods before conception and during pregnancy. Our diet was essentially Macrobiotic, which is dominantly vegetarian, going as high as fish on the food chain (and including eggs and some fermented dairy products). I personally have used soy foods, almost daily, for the last 30 years, with no obvious ill effect, so far.

My advice to clients about soy is this: Have no more than one serving of "cooling" soy foods per day (edame, tofu or soymilk) unless you have a "heated" condition. Have all the miso, tamari and tempeh that you like. I tend not to recommend soy protein isolate powder any more, since it is a mass-produced slurry and seldom available in an organic form. Even though many of the studies that show health benefits were done with soy protein isolate, I see it as a supplement rather than a food. Say what you want about tofu, at the very least we know that it has been safely consumed for centuries, by men, women and children.

The caveat is how well do you digest soy? Generally, if you eat soy foods and get gas and/or indigestion, it is not beneficial for you. Another clue is your blood type. Types A and AB tend to digest it most efficiently and gain the greater benefit. And, trust your taste buds. I like tofu and soymilk, as well as the fermented forms, and I feel satisfied after eating them. My body likes soy foods and digests them well, so I shall continue to enjoy them.

CLOSING

By understanding the basics of when and how to use protein, fats and carbs, we attain the beginning of designing the optimal diet. Adding to that, the knowledge of good quality protein, bad quality carbohydrates (refined) and the ugly fats (over-heated and hydrogenated vegetable oils), we further define our diet. To my way of thinking, the final touch is to incorporate your blood type ("The Blood Type Diet": see Chapter Six), and to eat what grows within 500 miles of where you live, and in season (or naturally preserved).

CHAPTER THREE

CHOOSING A "GREEN" DRINK

The popularity of the so-called "green" drinks has lead to an explosion of these products in the marketplace. Once again, we can find ourselves overwhelmed by choices, and the ensuing marketing campaigns. In this chapter, I will attempt to simplify it a bit in order to aid you in picking a green product, should you feel you the need for one.

WHY BUY A GREEN DRINK?

Why indeed, would you need one? The long and short of it is: do you eat 5 to 7 servings of fruits and vegetable daily? These green drink mixes are marketed as an alternative to real food, and while that may not be 100% true, it is pretty tricky to get in 7 servings of fruits and veggies daily. We want these foods for a number of reasons, but most importantly for antioxidants, fiber and to alkalize our bodies.

Antioxidants, which are found at much higher levels in berries than vegetables, can help protect us from premature aging, cancer and many other diseases. Fiber intake is critical to preventing bowel cancer, and for stabilizing insulin levels, which both prevents diabetes and excessive weight gain. (Not to mention, just keeping the bowels moving regularly.) And, keeping our bodies more alkaline than acidic is the key to general health and well-being, and is especially important for preventing cancer and osteoporosis.

When you purchase a green drink it will contain antioxidants, trace minerals and other subtle nutrients not found in vitamin pills, and as well, you will get the pigment chlorophyll, which is what makes something green. Chlorophyll alkalizes the body and is also an amazing detoxifier, cleansing the bowel, blood and liver. It also helps to build red blood cells, and so is important to maintain physical energy and vitality.

WHAT'S MISSING

These drinks are usually taken in the morning, often providing an energizing alternative to coffee, but when substituting them for food, there are a couple of things missing that we should be aware of.

FIBER

You are not going to get an appreciable amount of fiber in a green drink. So, if that is something that you feel the need for, you can add a fiber mix to your morning regimen. I often add in a tablespoon of defatted flax powder, along with a teaspoon of "Inulin" (derived from chicory) to my morning shake, or even to my oatmeal. This gives me the mixed benefits of both soluble fiber (Inulin) and insoluble fiber (flax).

Soluble fiber serves as a "pre-biotic", encouraging the growth of colonies of friendly bacteria (probiotics) in the intestinal tract, and helps to keep cholesterol in check. Insoluble fiber works as roughage, keeping us regular and cleaning the intestines. And the "lignans", found in flax meal (de-fatted, so as to avoid the potential for the delicate oils to go rancid), help to pull hormone-mimicking chemicals ("xenoestrogens") from the body.

When adding extra fiber to the diet, it is best to start off slowly (1/2 the recommended amount) and gradually work your way up to the desired dosage. Too much fiber, too fast, will cause flatulence in those not accustomed to it

PROTEIN

Now, if you call your green drink "breakfast," you are also not going to get any protein, which I didn't mention as a benefit of fruits and vegetables, since they don't contain much. But it is critical to have protein in the morning if you are middle-aged or older, if you are an athlete, or if you have blood sugar issues. As mentioned in the previous chapter, by middle age, and when under extra physical stress, the body will lose muscle mass if it is not given protein in the morning. Protein, as well as fiber, also keeps insulin levels stable. Some drink mixes do add fiber and protein to their greens and/or berries, providing a better balance for those who do not eat in the mornings.

WHAT TO LOOK FOR IN A GREEN DRINK

There are two things to look at when choosing a green drink. First, look at the list of ingredients, which are in descending order, from most to least. There are two general categories of these drinks; those in which lecithin is the first ingredient, and those generally more expensive ones, which do not contain lecithin.

Lecithin, derived from soybeans, is a wonderful substance with the ability to improve short-term memory, and the function of cleaning fatty deposits off of the liver and out of the arteries. It is, however, a relatively cheap substance to purchase on its own, which is why the more expensive products don't contain it. If you would like the benefits of lecithin, but not in your drink mix, it can be purchased in capsule form.

The trick here is not to buy "lecithin" capsules, but instead look for "Phosphatidylcholine" (PS), which is commonly referred to as "triple-strength lecithin." Clinical studies that are loosely translated to "lecithin" are actually done with PS, and since the effective dose is 3 capsules of PS, you would need 9 capsules of lecithin to get the same effect. Lecithin may also be purchased in granule form, which is added to shakes or breakfast cereal (or yogurt, etc) by the tablespoon.

The higher-end green products give you more of the actual fruits and vegetables along with the concentrated cereal (wheat, barley, etc) grass juices, rather than the cheaper whole grass concentrates. The ground whole grasses have a gritty texture, which negatively affects the "mouth-feel" of the drink, without actually adding any appreciable fiber. Products that use concentrated grass juice (where the fibrous parts have been removed) have a smoother texture and go down easier. Also, an equal amount of grass juice will have more beneficial nutrients than a comparable amount of ground grass.

Other elements found in green drinks often include herbal concentrates and super foods, such as royal jelly, bee pollen and algae. If the focus is on fruits and vegetables, be sure that they are organic, as non-organic fruit especially, can be high in pesticides.

TOO MANY INGREDIENTS

The other questionable thing about the mixed greens products, aside from what they don't have, is the amount of ingredients in that combination. The oriental approach to diet is two-fold: eat what grows within 500 miles of where you live, because only in our recent history could a human travel further than that, and because food is attuned to its environment, and eat simply to keep your thinking simple. This does not mean that it keeps you simple-minded, but rather, that we Westerners tend to already be overstimulated, and to think too much, often to the point of anxiety and sleep disorders.

A product that combines 30 different substances, from different areas of the world, into one meal, is far from simple. Also, this type of product may include a number of herbs that are generally best taken for short periods in order to prevent a tolerance from building up (e.g. Milk Thistle), lessening their specific effectiveness. As well, if you are prone to allergies, which one of the 30-some ingredients is the one that is problematic for you? And, of course, if one product has 30 ingredients then the next one on the block has to one-up them by having 40 ingredients, and so on.

How about one ingredient? These substances all have different properties. Grasses are considered "yang" and "grounding" because they grow in the earth. This would be good for vegetarians. Algae such as spirulina and chlorella, are considered more "yin" because they grow in water, and would generally be better for meat eaters, who already have a yang diet. Spirulina is considered a "damp" food in Chinese medicine, and so should be avoided in excess by those with candida yeast problems. Barley grass and chlorella are both good for "kidney essence" (in the Chinese system), which is our storehouse of vitality, and so are both very good for the aged. Chlorella is a master detoxifier, especially of chemicals and mercury.

The point here is that sometimes it is a good idea to get a sense of one substance, to see how our body likes it, or to get enough of it for a therapeutic action. For example, with chlorella, if I have mercury fillings there would not be enough of it available for removing mercury, when the chlorella is only one of 30 ingredients in the serving. Perhaps, in the damp of West Coast winters, I would be better off with the drying tendencies of barley or wheat grass, whereas in the summer I can take more spirulina, because the season is dry, and thus the damp qualities of the algae are not an issue.

I have said it before and I will say it again: "more is not better." When I help someone choose a greens product I will point out these considerations, and emphasize that since the serving sizes are generally roughly the same, more ingredients just equals less of everything. I will steer them to a product with less ingredients, rather than more.

I suggest one look for (or concoct) a product where the algae are balanced by a similar amount of cereal grass juices, and where the fruits used could be found growing in an environment, similar to where you live. A green drink like this, with added fiber and protein, essentially turn the mix into a meal (even more so, if you add a tablespoon of nutritional oil to it). It's not rocket science, quite the opposite; it is just a matter of keeping it simple.

CHAPTER FOUR

THE MAGIC OF GREEN TEA

In this chapter we are going to review some of the benefits of what amounts to a "superfood": good, old-fashioned green tea. Becoming a frequent drinker of green tea (or using a quality supplement) is perhaps one of the most valuable things you can do for your overall health.

The herb "camellia sinensis" is commonly known as "tea", and has been shown in studies from around the world to provide a wide range of health benefits. Tea, infused from the leaves of this plant, is the most popular beverage in the world, next only to water. While black tea also has some health benefits, the darker the tea the more processing it has undergone, and the more the benefits diminish, as the antioxidants are lost.

In keeping with this principle, the white tea leaf has the highest level of benefit, followed by green tea, and downhill from there. White tea is green tea picked at an earlier stage in its growth and, while more powerful than green tea, is also more expensive. "When the two teas are exposed to viruses, fungi, and staphylococcus bacteria, white tea killed 80% of the sample, while green tea killed only 60%"(Alternative Medicine, Sept./2004). For convenience, I will refer to green tea instead of mentioning both green and white. Though their benefits are similar, with white tea being somewhat stronger, almost all studies, both population and otherwise, are based on green tea.

These benefits of green tea are derived from the "polyphenols," which are a class of antioxidant components found in the tea leaf. Numerous animal, human and laboratory studies have demonstrated significant anti-carcinogenic, anti-inflammatory and anti-microbial properties. Let's have a closer look at some of these attributes.

ANTIOXIDANT

In experimental studies, the polyphenols found in green tea have shown greater antioxidant activity than both vitamin C and vitamin E. Polyphenols are a unique class of bioflavonoids that are found throughout the diet. The richest sources are the blue, red and purple colored fruits and plants, as the polyphenols are found in the pigments, and especially in the skins, of such foods. Thus the richest sources of polyphenols are found in berries, grapes and wine, but are also found in appreciable amounts in dark beer, coffee, chocolate and olive oil. Science strongly supports the position that polyphenols contribute to the prevention of cancer, heart disease and osteoarthritis.

The most important of the polyphenol compounds found in green tea are the catechins, in particular EGCG (epigallocatechin), which has been shown to have 200 times more antioxidant activity than vitamin E. As well as exerting its own antioxidant activity, green tea has been shown to elevate the body's antioxidant protective system, by raising levels of the enzymes "super oxide dismutase" (SOD) and glutathione (peroxidase).

ANTI-BACTERIAL

Green tea has the ability to kill bacteria and this has served humans well in two areas: the mouth and the digestive system. Catechins will bind with nitrogen and sulfur in the mouth, eliminating the cause of bad breath (as opposed to just masking it, as with most mouthwashes). Green tea also blocks the attachment of bacteria to teeth, protecting against cavities. The American Society for Microbiology stated in 2003: "Studies conducted at Pace University have indicated that green tea extract has an adverse effect on bacteria that cause strep throat, dental cavities and other infections."

EGCG also protects against digestive and respiratory infections, and encourages acidophilus ("good" bacteria) colonization while regulating bowel movements. Catechins in general are known to completely kill cholera viruses and E. Coli bacteria, further protecting the digestive system.

ANTI-CARCINOGENIC

In the parts of the world where green tea is regularly consumed, the incidence of solid tumor cancers, such as breast, lung and gastrointestinal cancers, is demonstrably lower. In fact the Linus Pauling Institute, in March 2003, went so far as to state that, "Green and white teas exert significant protective effects in experimental animal models of skin, lung, esophageal, gastric, hepatic, small intestinal, pancreatic, colon, bladder and mammary cancer."

This anti-cancer effect is the result of the polyphenols blocking the formation of cancer-causing compounds, as well as effectively detoxifying or trapping carcinogens. Research at the Medical College of Georgia showed that compounds in green tea selectively induced cell death in oral cancer cells, while ignoring normal cells. The authors of this study concluded that green tea could inhibit, delay or even reverse, oral cancer. Their position is supported by the population studies from China, where it was observed that Chinese oral cancer rates are half that of North America, even though the smoking rates are three times higher in China (Vancouver Sun, Jan 12/02).

ANTI-INFLAMMATORY

Green Tea contains natural COX-2 inhibitors that can help reduce inflammation and which, unlike pharmaceutical COX-2 inhibitors, have no side effects. Furthermore, one of the major factors in the progression of osteoarthritis is cartilage destruction, and compounds found in green tea (EGCG and ECG) can block the enzyme that destroys cartilage. Sheffield University in the United Kingdom has already taken out a patent for the use of EGCG in treating osteoarthritis. ("Catechins from Green Tea inhibit Bovine and Human Cartilage Proteoglycan and Type II Collagen Degradation in vitro." Journal of Nutrition 132; 2002)

Because inflammatory mechanisms in the body are at the root of many diseases besides arthritis, including Alzheimer's disease, heart disease and certain forms of cancer, the benefits of naturally reducing inflammation are very broad (as we shall see in a forthcoming chapter).

HEART PROTECTOR

Regular consumption of green tea protects against heart disease and stroke, due to the mechanisms of catechins. Aside from the cardiovascular benefits of its antioxidant and anti-inflammatory abilities, green tea can help prevent lipoprotein oxidation (leading to "bad" cholesterol) and platelet clumping. Furthermore, the component EGCG activates the release of nitric oxide (NO) in the endothelial cells lining the blood vessels. This in turn relaxes the smooth muscles within the blood vessel walls, dilating them and improving blood flow. (As a side note, this is, in part, the function of Viagra, so green tea may provide long term benefit to ones' sex life, as well.) Along with improved vascular circulation, EGCG further reduces the inflammatory chemicals (cytokines) linked to atherosclerosis and heart disease, preventing vascular blockage and the ensuing stroke or heart attack.

NEURO-PROTECTIVE

Neuro-degenerative diseases, which are also tied to inflammation, appear to be reduced and prevented by regular green tea consumption. "There is now a large body of scientific evidence... demonstrating that certain natural compounds, such as catechins from green tea, improve age-related cognitive decline, and are neuroprotective in animal models of Parkinson's disease, Alzheimer's disease, stroke, Huntington's disease, amyotrophic lateral sclerosis (ALS) and other brain diseases." – Dr. Frank L. Bradford, University of Buffalo School of Medicine & Biomedical Sciences (Quoted in Life Extension, April 2008.)

Even when you give young, healthy rats green tea catechins for a long period, they show better memory and learning abilities over time, than the control rats that did not receive the supplementation. Just so you know that it's not all rat studies, we have a population study done on over a thousand Japanese, aged 70 or older. Those who drank at least one cup of green tea per day showed a "38% decrease in cognitive impairment," compared to those who drank coffee, black tea, or 3 or less cups of green tea in a week (American Journal of Clinical Nutrition; Feb 2006).

ANTI-STRESS

Green tea contains the amino acid L-Theanine (almost exclusively found in the tea plant), a powerful nutrient that can help to reduce stress levels. Most of the research into L-Theanine is being done in the area of stress reduction without drowsiness. While green tea does contain some caffeine (though far less than coffee, and less than black tea), it has been noted that green tea is very calming, for most people. This is because L-Theanine, in small amounts, is an antagonist to caffeine, so even though you are getting the positive effects of caffeine, in terms of staying alert, you are not getting the negative side effects associated with caffeine, such as jitters and nausea. Other current areas of research on L-Theanine include using it in isolated form as an alternative to Ritalin (for Attention Deficit children, with or without hyperactivity), controlling blood pressure, and sharpening mental acuity and concentration.

IMMUNE SUPPORT

Researchers have also found that L-Theanine may strengthen the body's immune system response, when fighting off infection. The findings were first discovered in laboratory cell cultures and then verified in a small human study. Scientists compared the immune system strength of men and women before and after they started to drink tea. A control group drank coffee instead. The study showed that those people who drank 5 to 6 small cups of black tea per day were better equipped to prevent infection. The anti-viral effect of green tea (stronger than that of black tea), has been shown to be much more effective when the caffeine is present, than that of decaffeinated teas (Brigham and Women's Hospital; April/03).

THERMOGENICS

As well as being a safe weight loss aid, gently speeding up the metabolism (which is what "thermogenic" means), green tea also stabilizes blood sugar levels, which helps to prevent the storage of carbohydrates as fat and to prevent diabetes. One study measured the effect of green tea on energy expenditure in healthy men who took it 3 times per day. The study concluded, that the men taking this extract burned 266 more calories per day than those in the placebo group ("Relationship Among Habitual Tea Consumption Percentage Body Fat and Body Fat Distribution"; Obesity Research II: 2003).

It is a little known fact that the average Westerner does not get the fat-burning properties from green tea, due to how we brew it. The standard 3 to 5 minute steep may provide the antioxidant benefits, but in order to get the thermogenic properties out of the tea, it requires at least 30 minutes steeping, under heat. This is the way the Asian cultures brew tea: leaving it on the stove, under heat, for long periods. Most of us find the result to be too bitter for our tastes. One way around this, is to drink "Matcha", the form of tea where you whisk the finely ground small leaves into liquid, in effect eating the whole leaf. The other option is to use a green tea supplement.

BLOOD SUGAR CONTROL

Glucose metabolism in healthy subjects has been shown to improve with daily green tea consumption. And, in a large population study, those who consumed 4 or more cups of green tea daily showed a reduced risk of diabetes, compared to those who did not consume tea (Journal of the American College of Nutrition; Oct 2005).

Scientists are not exactly sure how green tea controls high blood sugar, as the process probably involves a few different hormonal and metabolic functions. But, based on animal studies, we do know that the component EGCG regulates genes involved with glucose metabolism and insulin regulation (Journal of Agriculture & Food Chemistry; Jul 2007). In these studies, EGCG essentially mimicked the functions of insulin, and as well, reduced cholesterol and triglyceride accumulation in the hearts of diabetic rats. This strongly implies that green tea in one form or another, may prevent, or reduce, the disabling side effects that accompany diabetes caused by damage to the blood vessels in the eyes, heart, kidneys and limbs, as well as other organs.

GREEN TEA SUPPLEMENTS

The average cup of green tea provides approximately 80 to 110mg of polyphenols. This varies based on the type of green tea used and the brewing technique. A cup of green tea can contain from 40 to 80mg of caffeine, again depending on how long it has been brewed. (For comparison, a cup of coffee contains about 100 to 200mg of caffeine.)

Supplementing with green tea products can be a good idea in order to reap the full benefits, since it is difficult for all but the most dedicated drinker to obtain the 5 or more cups per day, where the greatest benefit is shown. But, when choosing a supplement it is a good idea to remember that many of these benefits have been established through "population studies." This is based on observing and tracking cultures that use green tea as a major part of their beverage intake. Certainly, laboratory experiments have shown great benefit to be derived from isolated components (EGCG for example), but these benefits are usually demonstrated in petri dishes or on rats.

Many products will claim to be equivalent to countless cups of tea, but they are only equal in a limited number of components. As is common in the West, we try to reduce a herb or food to its drug-like, isolated "effective" component, then claim that it is the same as using the whole substance. Let's look at a few examples of why this is a flawed approach when considering green tea.

TAMPERING WITH NATURE

Some green tea products begin by removing the caffeine, yet recent studies, from Rutgers University, concluded that caffeine in green tea was important to activating the herb's anti-tumor properties (Beyond Aspirin: The Cox-2 Medical Revolution; T. Newmark and P. Schulick; 2000; Hohm Press). As well, "study findings indicate that…caffeinated green and black tea are more effective as anti-viral agents than decaffeinated green and black teas" (American Society for Microbiology; May 20, 2003).

The next level of tampering is standardization, which usually involves chemical solvents to get consistent concentrated levels of an "active" compound. The most common compound chosen, due to having the most anti-tumor activity, is the polyphenol EGCG. But, in 1998 Japanese scientists showed that the "non-phenolic fraction (those components that are not polyphenols) has potent suppressive activities against tumor promotion" ("Beyond Aspirin"). This confirms that it is a mix of all the compounds found naturally occurring in tea, working in unison, that do what the population studies have indicated. Thus, when choosing a supplement search for one that is a complex structure of the concentrated whole plant, and not one that trades off unexplored compounds for "scientifically valid" ones.

Finally, when choosing to supplement with green tea products, remember that a pill is also different from a beverage. When drinking the tea we get three main benefits that are missing when swallowing a pill. As mentioned above, green tea has a strong reputation for killing bacteria that causes bad breath, cavities and other oral infections, and has been demonstrated to lower mouth cancer rates. These benefits only accrue when the tea runs through the mouth, and so there is a strong advantage to a liquid green tea concentrate that may be taken straight or added to water (or other beverages).

WARNINGS

The medical profession warns that green tea, as a supplement and beverage, can have an adverse effect on certain medications. Before using green tea on a consistent basis, consult with a health professional if you are using penicillin-type antibiotics, beta-blockers, blood thinning medications, anti-anxiety or anti-depressant drugs. Green tea can increase the effectiveness of some drugs, making the recommended dose too powerful, and reduce the effectiveness of others (particularly lithium).

The consumption of green tea at high temperatures, as is done in many traditional Asian cultures, has been linked to increased risk of esophageal cancer therefore tea should be imbibed at a moderate, or low temperature (in other words, it should not burn your mouth).

CHAPTER FIVE

ADRENAL EXHAUSTION

"Energy can be neither created nor destroyed, only transformed:

First Law of Thermo-dynamics

In modern times, adrenal exhaustion is rampant and responsible, in part, for a host of ailments, including two of particular concern: hormonal imbalance (in both women and men) and fat storage around the abdomen (the most dangerous kind). Let's look at why modern living is so hard on our adrenal glands, and what we can do about it.

Lack of energy is a common complaint these days, however, when one goes seeking "energy", it is good to remember the old adage: "There is no such thing as a free lunch." That cup of coffee, can of pop, cigarette or "fat-burning" pill, will give you temporary energy, but you are going to pay for it later. This is because stimulants work by stealing energy from elsewhere, to provide it when you demand it. When that energy wears off there is a crash, and your base energy level will be lower than it was when you first ingested the stimulant.

The area of your body that is most abused by the use of stimulants is the adrenal glands, which also happen to be your first line of defense against stress. The adrenals are involved in many functions essential to well being. These include regulating heart rate, blood pressure, respiration and digestion, as well as producing some of the sex hormones. But, from an "energy" perspective, the most important thing adrenal glands do, is regulate our "fight or flight" response.

ADRENAL ABUSE

In our distant past, a danger signal would jump-start the adrenals to mobilize the resources of the body for immediate activity, so that we could fight or flee the danger. In modern life, most of the danger signals must be ignored. When your boss yells at you, you can't hit him and you can't run away. All day long, every day, the stressors are triggering our adrenal response: bad drivers (don't get me started on bad drivers), family problems, job worries, sirens and high or low level noise in the work place, to name but a few.

Constant stress combined with stimulant use (remember that even sugar has stimulant properties), will finally exhaust the adrenal glands so that they can no longer provide the energy you need, when you need it. They can also malfunction in the direction of producing too much energy when you don't need it (i.e. anxiety and panic attacks). Adrenal exhaustion can contribute to the development of hypoglycemia, insomnia (indicated especially when one wakes in the middle of the night), depression, allergies, menopausal symptoms, circulatory problems, and immune malfunction. Low energy, of course, is the result of adrenal exhaustion, and at its extreme can lead to conditions of physical exhaustion, such as chronic fatigue syndrome.

CORTISOL AND DHEA

One major side effect of adrenal exhaustion is the ensuing tendency for levels of the stress hormone "cortisol" to spike. High cortisol levels elevate blood pressure and lead to abdominal fat storage, considered the most dangerous fat, because it is the type of fat that can produce more fat. When people are looking at a weight loss plan, I always encourage them to make sure they have taken care of their adrenals.

Hormonal imbalances, especially menopause and andropause (the male version), are due to reduced DHEA (dehydroepiandrosterone,) production in the body. During such an imbalance, high estrogen in a woman and low testosterone in a male, are both linked to excessive weight-gain. As we age, the ovaries and gonads lose their ability to produce the sex hormones. It is then up to the adrenal glands to take up the slack, by producing extra DHEA. This "mother" hormone will in turn produce estrogen, progesterone and testosterone, in optimal amounts for each body. All three sex hormones are required for both genders, but in varying ratios.

A note to Canadians: DHEA is illegal to possess in Canada, without a prescription, since it has been classified as a steroid hormone. It is a building block for steroid (i.e. sex) hormones, but as a supplement is considered relatively safe when used at low dosage levels. I have, however, seen a woman raise her DHEA levels by 20% over two months by using a good adrenal rebuilding formula. (Hormone tests, using saliva, are now commonly available through doctors and pharmacists.)

NUTRITIONAL SUPPORT

Proper adrenal support must include a good diet. Try to avoid drinking coffee: black tea is a better choice and green tea an even better choice (as we saw in Chapter Four). As much as possible, one should avoid refined carbohydrates, including sugars, fruit juices, breads, pastries, white rice, potatoes and pasta (unless it is whole grain). Eat on a regular basis (three good meals daily) with healthy snacks in between meals (whole fruits, nuts and seeds) with an emphasis on protein, vegetables and complex carbohydrates (whole grains, yams and sweet potatoes).

As well, certain nutrients are required to maintain adrenal health, including vitamins B-5, B-6 and C, and the minerals Magnesium and Zinc. Try to get at least 500mg to 1000mg of vitamin C with each meal, and include at least 20mg of vitamin B-6 (along with the rest of the B vitamins) at least once a day, along with some zinc (15mg for women to 30mg for men). For serious adrenal rebuilding we add a vitamin B-5 (Pantothenic Acid) supplement (250mg three times daily, with food) and a Magnesium supplement (400 to 600mg daily in divided doses).

Once we've fulfilled our nutritional requirements, we turn to the herbal-supportives.

Certain herbs known as "adaptogens," support organisms in dealing with all stressors: emotional, mental and physical. These agents do the most to rebuild exhausted adrenal glands, and many of them are combined in "Adrenal" or "Energy" formulas. Such a formula should be used for at least a month, along with the dietary advice and nutritional support mentioned above. Among the best-researched adaptogens are: Ashwagandha, Fo Ti, Royal Jelly, Schizandra, Siberian Ginseng (Eleutherococcus) and Rhodiola Rosea.

Here is a quick look at some of that research. A Swedish study looked at "a fixed combination of three genuine extracts of Eleutherococcus senticocus, Schisandra chinensis and Rhodiola rosea" and concluded that, "adaptogens increase tolerance to stress in our model combination of physical and emotional stresses" (Phytomedicine. 2009 Jun). A further Swedish study, by the same institute (SHI Research and Development), reviewed clinical trials of the same three adaptogens and had this to say: "Strong scientific evidence is available for Rhodiola rosea extract, which improved attention, cognitive function and mental performance in fatigue and in chronic fatigue syndrome. Good scientific evidence has been documented in trails (mediated pathways) in which Schisandra chinensis and Eleutherococcus senticocus increased endurance and mental performance in patients with mild fatigue and weakness (Curr Clin Pharmacol. 2009 Sep)."

For those who are under day-to-day stress I suggest using L-Theanine, the amino acid derived from green tea. It will reduce your stress response both quickly and safely (150mg to 300mg; and can be used as a sleep aid, at higher dosage levels: 300 to 450mg).

A CLOSER LOOK AT ADAPTOGENS

ASHWAGANDHA (Withania Somifera)**:** This herb grows in India and is commonly used to treat fatigue and general debility. It has properties that make it useful in sexual support formulas, having been shown to reduce the frequency of premature ejaculation and to increase sexual stamina. Ashwagandha is especially good for physical activity, as it gives long-lasting energy with no "crash," and is now commonly used in the sports and fitness fields. It also prevents memory loss and mental deterioration, and animal studies have found it to be more effective than hydrocortisone for controlling inflammation, in cases of arthritis and carpal tunnel syndrome.

FO TI (Polygonum Multiflorum)**:** Used for centuries by the Chinese, this herb is considered a tonic for fertility, longevity and rejuvenation. Fo Ti, also known as Ho Shou Wu, tones the entire glandular system (especially the liver and kidneys) along with the adrenals. Fo Ti is known to promote stabilization of blood sugar levels, and is often prescribed to return gray hair to its original color. Traditionally used as a calming herb by the Chinese, especially for insomnia and nightmares, it has also been shown in lab tests to reduce cholesterol and triglycerides. Believed to purify the blood, Fo Ti is also used to treat infertility, impotence, vaginal discharges, infectious diseases and angina. This herb can be a little heating to the system, and so is generally combined with cooling herbs, such as Royal Jelly or North American ginseng, in order to balance out that tendency.

RHODIOLA ROSEA: Native to the mountains of Asia and Europe, Rhodiola has been used there for centuries to fight fatigue and restore energy. Rhodiola supports the central nervous system, improving memory, learning and attention, while reducing stress. It has been shown to regulate the sex hormones in both genders, to support thyroid function, and to function as an antioxidant and anti-carcinogen.

ROYAL JELLY: This miracle food from the bee hive contains every known nutrient – all vitamins, minerals, amino acids, enzymes and essential fatty acids – providing its energy from compact synergistic nutrition. Royal jelly is particularly high in Pantothenic Acid (B-5), a critical nutrient for adrenal health. An interesting thing about Royal Jelly is how it affects the longevity of the bees. The life span of a bee is, on average, about 6 weeks, except for the queen bee, who lives for nearly 6 years, while producing thousands of eggs. The queen bee is genetically no different from the other bees; she just won the fight to determine who the new queen will be. The difference is that other bees only get Royal Jelly when they are infants, while the queen lives off of it her whole life. This is one reason why the Chinese have associated it with health and longevity for centuries.

SCHIZANDRA (Schisandra chinensis)**:** A traditional Chinese herb that works synergistically with Siberian Ginseng as an anti-stress adaptogen, Schizandra also provides many other benefits. These include improved digestion, increased circulation, enhanced immune function, and increased stamina and physical performance. Schizandra berries (the part of the plant utilized) are widely used in Asia to treat liver diseases (especially cirrhosis and hepatitis) and, since in oriental medicine the liver is related to the eyes, to increase visual acuity and range of vision. To Western science, Schizandra's benefits to the liver are proven in laboratory studies that show its ability to increase the production of glutathione in the liver. It can also block the production of the inflammatory fatty acid "arachidonic acid" in the body, serving, in part, as an anti-inflammatory. Schizandra has also been used traditionally to treat insomnia, restless legs, depression and excessive sweating.

SIBERIAN GINSENG (Eleutherococcus senticosus)**:** This adaptogen, native to Siberia, is not a true ginseng, and is no longer allowed to be referred to as such in the U.S. (due to the work of the ginseng grower's lobby), where it is known by its latin name, Eleutherococcus. An excellent adrenal re-builder, Siberian Ginseng has a long history of use for mental and physical exhaustion. Because it is not a ginseng, per se, it is safe to be used by either gender over a long period of time. True ginseng requires a little more finesse to be used safely. "Red" ginseng (Chinese or Korean) is heating to the body and can raise blood pressure, or worsen "hot flashes" due to menopause, whereas "white" ginseng (North American) has the opposite effect of cooling the body. As such it could be used to alleviate those heated conditions. In either case, one should not use a red or white ginseng for longer than a month. Overheating or overcooling our body for too long, without the advice of a health professional, can lead to health problems.

Used traditionally for over 2000 years, Siberian Ginseng also has many modern applications as well. It helps the liver to detoxify radiation, chemicals and toxins, and is used to treat ADD and depression. Commonly used in the sports field because it reduces post-workout fatigue and muscle soreness, it has also been shown to reduce the rate of respiratory infection in professional athletes by 35%. Of value to both athletes and those trying to maintain a healthy bodyweight, is the ability of Siberian Ginseng to moderate the production of cortisol in the body. Cortisol is "catabolic" (muscle destroying), and Siberian Ginseng can deactivate cortisol before it causes damage to muscle tissue. Also used to treat chronic fatigue syndrome, reduced sex drive in men, autoimmune diseases, and lung and viral infections

A WORD ABOUT COFFEE

Many of us jump-start the day with a cup of coffee. This practice is, at the very least, debatable from the point of view of adrenal health, but all the worse when we call it breakfast. As mentioned earlier ("This is a Protein…"), by the time we approach middle age, our body starts displacing (i.e. eating) our muscle mass, if we don't have protein in the morning. But we get to keep the fat, and since muscle burns fat, the more muscle we lose over time, the harder it is to shake those extra pounds. Also, if we sweeten the coffee, we have added an insulin spike to the start of the day, leading to a roller coaster ride of blood sugar levels for the rest of the day.

If this is how you start your day, I suggest incorporating a protein into the morning routine. Personally, I often take a cup of almond or rice milk, add the remaining half of a mug of my coffee, a scoop of whey protein isolate, and some flax fiber and flax seed oil (1 tbsp). The fiber and oil slow down the transit time of the protein through the gut. This allows the shake to stick around long enough to constitute a meal. Aside from preserving muscle mass, whey protein enhances immune function and, like any protein, helps to keep your blood sugar levels stable. For those who just don't feel like eating in the mornings, this shake goes down fairly easily. At the very least, if the addition of fiber and oil doesn't sound appetizing, just mix a protein into your coffee. (Warning: whey protein is about the only one where this works well, as far as taste goes.)

Another technique that adds value to the morning coffee is the addition of either burdock or dandelion root. Add from a quarter to a half of a teaspoon of herb to the water, bring to a boil, and then pour over the grounds. Both of these herbs support liver function, help detoxify the blood and help stabilize blood sugar levels. Since they have a slightly bitter taste, they complement the coffee well.

It is important when purchasing coffee that it be organic. Since coffee is a Third World cash crop, it is usually heavily sprayed with pesticides. Also, grinding it fresh offers potential immune enhancing benefits that are lost when grounds are old (oils go rancid), or when it has been brewed an hour or more ago. You will notice that old coffee, that has been kept hot for a length of time, leaves an unpleasant taste in the mouth. At this point it is mildly toxic.

One seldom considered fact about coffee is that it raises stomach acid levels. For blood types with low stomach acid (Type A and Type AB), coffee taken after a meal can aid digestion, and even on an empty stomach is not too abrasive. For those with Type O blood (the most common blood type) who are pre-disposed to high stomach acid levels, coffee on an empty stomach can be an irritant, and even contribute to ulcer formation. Those with Type O blood should usually only take coffee following food, especially if they find it hard on their stomach.

In the health field, coffee is considered to be least damaging when it is taken black, rather than whitened and sweetened. French and espresso roasts have less caffeine but more acids, which are hard on the digestive tract. Also, coffee and espresso drinks that are not filtered through paper leave in compounds linked to raising blood cholesterol levels.

ADRENAL SUPPORT TIPS

Exercise: Physical exercise, when done in moderation, decreases the body's production of adrenaline in response to stress, and increases energy by improving the use of oxygen and nutrients in the body. Excessive exercise, however, can cause adrenal exhaustion.

Relax: Relaxation lowers the heart rate and blood pressure, bringing us into a state opposite to the stress response. Learning relaxation techniques, before finding yourself in the middle of stressful living, is your best defense, but even if your life is currently out of control, it's never too late. Options include biofeedback, breathing exercises, meditation, prayer, self-hypnosis and visualization. They are all powerful and proven methods for reducing stress. Regular massage or any bodywork modalities can also induce relaxation that lasts well beyond the treatment. Yoga, aikido and tai chi can raise beta-endorphin levels in the body (the feel good hormones) in just 30 minutes.

Take a nap: Mid-afternoon is when your blood sugar levels normally decline, and when many people naturally crave coffee or sweets. This time, between 1 and 4 pm, is traditional siesta time in many countries. If you are able to nap for 15 or 30 minutes, you will wake up refreshed and ready to go.

Reduce coffee intake: If you are suffering from weak adrenals, even one cup of coffee can whip your adrenals into a state of exhaustion. The most powerful energizing beverage next to coffee, without the side effects, is the South American herb "Yerba Mate," which has caffeine-like alkaloids. Black tea is the methadone of coffee users. It offers protection against stroke, and, switching from coffee to black tea will still fulfill some of your caffeine needs. A variety of herbal teas can gently energize you while supporting your adrenals. These include ginseng, ginger, lemon, licorice, peppermint and rooibos. Just the fragrances of lemon and peppermint are uplifting and energizing. Licorice is especially good for the adrenals, but may be contraindicated in the case of high blood pressure.

Get enough sleep: We should get a minimum of eight hours of sleep each night to feel rested. According to the teachings of Ayurvedic medicine, body cycles indicate that the most important time to sleep is between 10 pm and 6 am. This is when the body is programmed to slow down and repair itself.

Soak up the sun: Try to get at least one hour of outside daylight everyday. Exposure to the sun is essential to balancing melatonin, the hormone that regulates your circadian rhythms and sleep cycles. Melatonin deficiency can also lead to depression, poor concentration, impaired immune function and reduced sex drive. A little known fact is that exposure to electromagnetic fields will disrupt the body's production of melatonin. The worst culprits are desktop computers, new cars, electric blankets and clock radios (those that plug into the wall). We need at least 4 feet between them and us to be out of their field of influence.

C H A P T E R   S I X

CONTROLLING INFLAMMATION

In order to maintain health in the 21st Century, it becomes imperative that we look at inflammation in the body. Our inflammatory mechanisms are designed to heal and protect the body, and can save us from dying of infection or injury. Yet, when this response gets out of control and becomes chronic, it can also cause damage throughout the body. Pain may not be so obvious in brain inflammation, due to its lack of pain receptors, but the damage caused there can be a cause of Alzheimer's disease, depression and schizophrenia.

Other health issues linked to inflammation include the obvious arthritic conditions, but as well cardiovascular disease, fibromyalgia, psoriasis, Crohn's disease and colitis. Even diabetes and certain forms of cancer are being linked to long-term inflammation in the body. So, controlling inflammation, through diet and supplements, is a wise idea for all of us, not just those with obvious pain issues.

DIET

The primary dietary approach to controlling inflammation is to avoid foods that are acidifying (sugars, refined carbohydrates, alcohol, coffee, processed foods, excess red meat) and focus on those foods that are alkalizing (whole fruits and vegetables, legumes, seafood, mineral water, olive oil, green tea). Avoid over-consumption of foods high in arachidonic acid (beef, egg yolks, dairy), and junk foods cooked at extremely high temperatures (chips, fries, deep fried foods). Even over-cooked foods (especially barbequed, broiled, "browned" and fried), and leftover foods (three or more days old), will contribute to inflammation.

We know that fiber keeps us regular and helps lower high cholesterol levels. Now a new study (The "Seasonal Variation of Blood Cholesterol Levels Study") has found that "the likelihood of elevated C-reactive protein was 63% lower in participants in the highest quartile of total fiber intake than in participants in the lowest quartile."

C-reactive protein, found in the blood, is a benchmark of inflammation that indicates the onset of diseases that are inflammatory in nature. These include diabetes, heart disease, cancer and Alzheimer's disease. It is important when you get blood work done, that you ask for a C-reactive protein test, as it is a far more important indicator of your potential for heart disease than a cholesterol reading is.

The researchers are uncertain as to how fiber affects the C-reactive protein levels, but they have hypothesized that soluble fiber, which acts as a pre-biotic in the intestinal tract, may be increasing good bacteria and decreasing bad bacteria, thereby improving general health and preventing inflammation from occurring.

Another dietary-related cause of inflammation is uric acid crystals, which deposit in the joints, resulting in pain and swelling. This condition is commonly known as Gout, but uric acid also contributes to the pain caused by other arthritic conditions. Red meat is considered the main source of excessive uric acid, but other foods can also contribute to its build up in the body. These include shellfish, organ meats, rich fatty foods (cream, gravy, sauces), alcohol (red wine especially), baking yeast, herring, sardines, anchovies, and high levels of vitamin B3 (over 500mg daily). If you are eating high amounts of these foods, you may want to stop for a month or so, and see if your symptoms improve.

BLOOD TYPE DIET

It is well known that members of the nightshade family of plants (bell peppers, potatoes, tomatoes and eggplant) can aggravate arthritic conditions in susceptible people. It turns out that this susceptibility may be due mainly to our blood type.

As a nutritional consultant, I have over the years repeatedly seen a positive response from clients who follow the blood type diet, popularized by Dr. Peter D'Adamo, in his book "Eat Right 4 Your Type." The areas that have produced the most positive feedback have been inflammatory conditions (especially arthritis) and weight loss.

The key factor to the blood type diet is the concept of "lectins." These are a form of protein that functions as a type of glue, a way for organisms in nature to attach themselves to other organisms. These lectins are found in cells, bacteria, microbes and food, and if they are incompatible with your blood type antigen, they will settle in different organs and body systems. There they draw other cells to that region and clump the cells together where the body perceives them as foreign invaders and attacks them. This clumping, for example, could trigger irritable bowel syndrome if they settle in the intestines, cirrhosis if they settle in the liver, or arthritis if they settle in the joints.

LECTINS

Most lectins from food don't make it very far into the body, but about 5% of the lectins that we eat get into the bloodstream, where they react with blood cells. This only becomes a problem if your blood type is reactive to that particular lectin. A food containing a certain lectin can be beneficial for one blood type but problematic for another.

The scientific community generally has little use for the blood type theory, but must admit two things: lectins show up under a microscope, and certain blood types have more incident of certain diseases than other blood types. These facts, combined with years of feedback from Naturopaths, and individuals who have used this diet effectively for a number of ailments, suggests that science will eventually take a closer look at this theory. There are in fact studies done with rabbits where lectins, derived from lentils, are injected into their knee joint cavity, resulting in the development of arthritis, showing all the properties of rheumatoid arthritis.

The criticism immediately is that "we don't inject lentils into our bloodstreams and therefore this is an invalid test." What is generally unacknowledged in the medical system is the tendency of modern people toward a thinning of the lining of the intestinal tract. This is due in part to the prevalence of candida yeast overgrowth, caused mostly by excessive antibiotic use and birth control pills. The other main cause of a thinned intestinal lining, is the widespread deficiency of vitamins A and D (see Part One), both of which are required in high amounts to maintain and regenerate all internal mucosal membranes.

This deficiency has occurred since we have ceased eating the livers of animals (including fish and fowl), which were our primary sources of these nutrients. Add to that, the insufficient vitamin D received due to living in the Northern Hemisphere, and the use of sun-block, etc, and we have a recipe for disaster. Now, instead of 5% of the lectins migrating into the bloodstream, we have up to 15%, or more. At this point, we see why the Blood Type Diet becomes an important modern paradigm necessary to deal with many ailments, including autoimmune disorders.

Since rheumatism, in Western medicine, is considered to be an autoimmune condition, it is important to remember that the response to lectins, in the bloodstream of a sensitive person, looks like an anti-body response. This is easily mistaken for an autoimmune condition, and so I suggest that anyone with any autoimmune illness pay especially close attention to the blood type diet.

In order to be succinct, I will at this juncture simply state that for our purposes, detrimental lectins create an inflammatory response in the body. Since inflammatory mechanisms are now linked to most major diseases, it behooves us to seriously consider this approach as part of our total health package.

At this point one really needs to find out their blood type. It is not covered by your government medical services plan, unless you require surgery, but if you donate blood you can find out for free; or you can pay a doctor or naturopath for the test, which should only cost about $25. Then procure a copy of Dr. Adamo's book, and read the section on your blood type, paying specific attention to when "lectins" are mentioned. These particular foods should then be mostly eliminated from your diet, and only consumed on rare or special occasions.

Many people use glucosamine as a natural treatment for arthritic conditions, and with great success. Yet, it turns out that it may be effective because of lectin-blocking actions. It has been demonstrated that glucosamine binds very effectively to wheat germ lectins (wheat being a particularly aggravating food for type O's). It is very possible that glucosamine works by sacrificing itself, reacting with lectins, thereby neutralizing the lectins and preventing them from reacting with the inflamed tissue. Thus the benefits of glucosamine supplementation may be due, at least partially, to mimicking the effects of a low lectin diet.

INFLAMMATORY FOODS FOR EACH BLOOD TYPE

Following is a list of the foods that most contribute to inflammation, for each blood type (though it is not a complete list):

Type A Blood: Red meat (this is not due to lectins, but to a lack of stomach acid in this blood type), tomatoes, potatoes, bell peppers, white vinegar, whole milk products (fermented and cultured dairy products are okay in moderation), bananas and oranges.

Type B Blood: Chicken (eggs and turkey are okay), pork, shellfish, corn, wheat, rye, lentils, peanuts, sesame and sunflower seeds (and their oils), tomatoes and black pepper.

Type AB Blood: Red meat, chicken, shellfish, sesame and sunflower seeds (and oils), corn, bell peppers, bananas, oranges, black pepper and white vinegar.

Type O Blood: Wheat gluten (sprouted wheat and wheat grass are okay), milk products, corn, eggplant, lentils, and potatoes.

WEIGHT LOSS AND BLOOD TYPE

A little out of context but, since we are on the subject of the Blood Type Diet, I am going to segue briefly into the topic of weight loss, and how it relates to this diet. You may skip this part if it doesn't interest you, but, since it is about blood sugar regulation, it also applies to preventing diabetes and hypoglycemia.

The other main detrimental aspect of the wrong lectins, aside from inflammation, is their ability to spike insulin levels. This means that seemingly innocuous foods can be fattening. For example, for my blood type (AB), chickpeas (garbanzo beans) fall into this category, so for me humus is a fattening food and can contribute to blood sugar irregularities.

Over years of client feedback, I have found enough anecdotal evidence to support the idea that the blood type diet offers a good dietary guideline to support a weight loss program, and that it is helpful for most people. But not everyone: as with most approaches there are exceptions to the rule, and for some people following this "diet" just doesn't work for them.

Certain type A's are too big and physical to be comfortable on a vegetarian diet, and some type O's that I've known have personal philosophies that do allow them to eat meat. Both examples may, however, still gain benefit from avoiding the lectins detrimental to their types. Type A will know that he needs extra digestive fluids if he is going to digest meat well (more so as he ages), and type O now knows that her protein requirements are going to be higher than that of some other vegetarians.

Nonetheless, many people have indicated to me that a long-term commitment (at least a year) to these basic dietary precepts, has distinctly aided them in regulating their bodyweight effectively. In essence, they found that their basic average weight "set-point" had dropped. Following are the basic premises of the blood type diet as related to weight loss:

TYPE "O" BLOOD: This blood type comes from hunter-gatherer stock and requires a high protein intake. As a result, this type makes a poor vegetarian, being prone to health problems if they do not ensure an adequate amount of protein in their diet. Meats, seafood and a variety of vegetables aid in their weight loss, while wheat products, especially, slow down their metabolic rate.

TYPE "A" BLOOD: In contrast, type A will often get fat from a meat-based diet, and are genetically suited to a modified vegetarian diet, coming historically from agrarian stock. While animal proteins speed up type O's metabolic rate, it slows down that of the type A. This difference is based on the stomach acid levels of each type. Type O is genetically prone to high stomach acid, which allows for easy meat digestion, and type A generally has comparatively low stomach acid, and so does not digest meat well. Type A's will get away with more carbs in the diet than type O's, but still need to stick to complex carbs for optimal health and weight. These include whole grains, yams and sweet potatoes. Dairy foods also contribute to weight gain in type A's. Weight loss in type A's is aided by consuming good quality oils (flax and olive), vegetables and soy foods (if adequate iodine intake is included in the diet).

TYPE "B" BLOOD: Originally of nomad stock, type B's need to avoid wheat, corn, lentils and peanuts, all of which for them impede metabolic efficiency and cause hypoglycemia. Foods that encourage weight loss in type B's include meat, eggs and dairy products, as well as green vegetables. Unlike O's and A's, type B's possess the genetics to properly digest dairy products, though they must be consumed moderately to achieve a metabolic balance. It should be noted that chicken is highly detrimental to the overall health of type B's.

TYPE "AB" BLOOD: Blood type AB is a rare and historically recent blood type, a merging of both A (agrarian) and B (nomad) blood types. While they have type B's adaptation to meat consumption, they also have type A's low stomach acid, which makes it difficult for them to metabolize meat effectively. As well as meat being fattening for type AB's, they also share the same insulin reaction as B's do towards corn and wheat, but the A blood allows them to easily digest peanuts and lentils. Foods that encourage weight loss for AB's include seafood, soy products, dairy (ideally fermented) and green vegetables.

DIGESTIVE DISORDERS

A word to the wise about digestive disorders which may occur in blood types A and AB. Because these two blood types are genetically prone to low stomach acid levels, should any symptoms of heartburn or acid reflux occur, the very worst thing to do is take acid suppressants. These symptoms can be caused by either high stomach acid or low stomach acid and, nine times out of ten, for these two blood types, they are caused by low stomach acid.

The correct response should be to increase their stomach acid levels, in order to reverse the symptoms. This can be done by ingesting a tablespoon of apple cider vinegar, or lemon juice, mixed with a little water, before meals, or when the symptoms occur. If the symptoms worsen, then indeed, your acid levels are too high. If they improve, however, you can then acquire "Betaine HCL" (basically, stomach acid in a pill) capsules, to maintain digestive functions. Remember that this situation also occurs in the elderly, since as we age our stomach acid levels naturally decline.

As an experiment, try eliminating those foods detrimental to your blood type for a month, and see what kind of difference you notice in your health. You have got nothing to lose but your pain and excess body fat. For more information see Dr. D'Adamo's book or visit his website: www.dadamo.com

MEDICAL APPROACH

Aside from diet, there are many natural remedies for inflammation but, unfortunately, what is commonly offered to those in pain, by the medical profession, comes with a cost over and above the monetary one. Most frequently turned to are the "non-steroidal anti-inflammatory drugs" (NSAIDs). The most common side effects are stomach pain, indigestion, ulcers, gastric hemorrhage and kidney damage. U.S. statistics attribute over 40,000 hospital admissions and over 3,000 deaths involving elderly patients each year, due to the use of NSAIDs. And, this is when they are used as prescribed.

Next, we have the steroidal anti-inflammatory drugs, prescribed when the non-steroidal versions don't work. Common adverse reactions include gastrointestinal irritation and bleeding, suppression of immune function, susceptibility to infection, and edema. Ironically, while cortisone injections will effectively reduce pain and inflammation, they also destroy cartilage and connective tissue in the joints, a further contribution to the cause of the pain, in the long run.

The newest generation of drugs for treating inflammation, are known as COX (Cyclooxygenase) inhibitors. They inhibit COX 2, an enzyme in the body that speeds up the production of chemical messengers, called prostaglandins. When the activity of COX 2 is blocked, the inflammation is reduced. But, recently it has been discovered that, the drugs that inhibit COX 2 have been linked to a 50% increase in the risk of heart attack and stroke in users. These drugs also inhibit COX 1, which protects the lining of the stomach, leading to the side effects of worsening gastric ulcers, colitis, and dyspepsia. Natural COX 2 inhibitors do not cause side effects, since they selectively inhibit COX 2 but do not inhibit COX 1.

GLUCOSAMINE AND MSM

One of the primary ways to combat arthritic inflammation is to take a quality joint-support supplement. These will combine the proven connective tissue rebuilding properties of Glucosamine and MSM (Methylsulfonylmethane), along with other natural substances designed to reduce inflammation and pain.

Aside from glucosamine's ability to neutralize lectins, we know that it also stimulates the production of "glycosamino glycans," one of the key structural components of cartilage. Some glucosamine converts in the body into chondroitin sulfate and hyaluronic acid, both of which help to lubricate the joints. While many joint products include chrondroitin sulfate along with glucosamine, few people are aware that it is made from the trachea of cows, and thus may not be ideal for all consumers.

Glucosamine is available in two forms, the most commonly used being Glucosamine "Sulfate," which has the most research behind it. The other form is Glucosamine "Hydrochloride," which contains 20% more active glucosamine than the sulfate form. The hydrochloride form is more commonly used for treating dogs, and for people who get heartburn from glucosamine sulfate. Glucosamine is involved in the formation of tendons, ligaments, cartilage and synovial fluids.

MSM is a sulfur compound, found naturally occurring in the human body, and in many foods. MSM is a basic element essential to many structures and functions of the human body. It has been clinically proven to lessen the pain of osteoarthritis and rheumatoid arthritis, as well as bursitis, carpal tunnel syndrome, tendonitis, and sports injuries, which it does by inhibiting pain impulses along nerve fibers. Sulfur compounds also have natural anti-inflamma-tory properties, and MSM has also been used to treat allergies and skin conditions. MSM is not similar to sulfides, sulfites, or sulfa drugs, which many people are allergic to.

ANTI-INFLAMMATORY EFA's

Essential Fatty Acids increase the production of "good" prosta-glandins, those that help to reduce inflammation. The best of these are the Omega 3 fatty acids, which have been shown to dramati-cally reduce pain and inflammation. These can be added to the diet in the form of flaxseed oil, by the tablespoon, or fish oil, by the teaspoon (which being a pre-converted form of fatty acid, is much stronger and requires less volume than does flaxseed oil). One re-quires at least one to two spoon-fulls of either oil, per day, to aid in reducing inflammation. But, it must be said that the science is mostly behind fish oil, though theoretically the flax oil should be similarly effective.

If we look at capsules instead of liquid, then we need to obtain between 1200mg and 2600mg of total Omega 3's (add up the DHA and EPA listed on the label) to get into anti-inflammatory terri-tory. Mixed fish oils which utilize the smaller fish (anchovies and sardines), are fifty percent stronger than salmon oil capsules, and so require less to be effective. On the other hand, you might have noticed that anchovies and sardines are on the avoid list for those prone to gout, or uric acid build-up. While this may be more due to the protein in the fish than the oil, it is best to err on the side of caution and use oils from other fish if you have these conditions.

Some authors have suggested that salmon oil is preferable for treating arthritic conditions because it contains calcitonin (unlike other fish oils). This substance is used therapeutically to treat hy-percalcemia (an excess of calcium in the blood), which has lead some to conclude that it may also be capable of gradually washing calcification out of the joints. Another bonus to calcitonin is that it has been clinically shown to stimulate cartilage formation.

ANTIOXIDANTS

Antioxidants protect the joints from free radical damage, especially vitamin C and selenium, which are often found to be low in those who suffer from arthritic conditions. Vitamin C is also required for the synthesis of the connective tissue collagen within the body. Grape seed extract and Pycnogenol (pine bark extract) are both powerful antioxidants because they contain proanthocyanidins (PCO's), which increase intracellular levels of vitamin C, scavenge free radicals and inhibit the destruction of collagen. PCO's also help to treat circulatory disorders, and to prevent the release of compounds in the body that promote allergies and inflammation.

The mineral manganese increases levels of the antioxidant "Super Oxide Dismutase" (SOD) in the body, which helps to protect cells from damage and inflammation. In fact, SOD injections are routinely used in Europe as a treatment for inflammatory conditions, including arthritis. Other nutrients that combat inflammatory conditions include the minerals copper and silica. These both aid in the production of collagen (part and parcel of healthy tendons, ligaments and cartilage) and other connective tissues. As with all degenerative diseases, basic nutritional supplementation is essential to lay the groundwork, upon which the more specific treatments can be built.

SILICA

Now, a few words about the trace mineral Silica which, even though it is not an anti-inflammatory, per se, does have an important role to play. As we saw in Part One, Silica is a key nutrient in maintaining and restoring the health and resiliency of our hair, skin, bones, teeth and connective tissue.

Dr. A. Charnot, who has researched degenerative tissue and joint diseases, discovered that a deficiency of silica often accompanies such conditions. Silica's ability to enhance connective tissue has made it effective in the treatment of muscle-skeletal disorders, including arthritis and rheumatism. It is a building block for connective tissues such as elastin, collagen and mucopolysaccharides. Silica also stimulates chrondroblasts to deposit chondroitin sulphate and hyaluronic acid into the cartilage matrix, and will improve the effectiveness of glucosamine.

PROTEOLYTIC ENZYMES

All protein-digesting (proteolytic) enzymes have a secondary function of being anti-inflammatory, if there is no protein present for them to digest. When used for this purpose they are either taken on an empty stomach, or are "enteric-coated", which prevents them from being released into the stomach, where they might be used up digesting protein. The proteolytic enzymes most often prescribed for treating inflammation, are bromelain (from pineapple), pancreatin (from pig pancreas) and serratia peptidase (cultivated either from silkworm enzymes or aspergillus, the fungal strain used to produce "plant-based" digestive enzymes). We will look at the two not derived from dead animals (personal bias).

There are three therapeutic areas of use for proteolytic enzymes. First and most commonly, they are used as a natural alternative to pharmaceutical anti-inflammatory drugs to treat conditions of inflammation and pain. This includes osteoarthritis, rheumatism, carpal tunnel syndrome, tendonitis, sports injuries and post-operative swellings. Next, they are used as a treatment for respiratory tract diseases, including bronchial asthma, bronchitis and sinusitis. Finally, proteolytic enzymes are used to treat conditions involving arterial plaque build-up, which include atherosclerosis, varicose veins and phlebitis (vein inflammation).

BROMELAIN

Bromelain is often overlooked as an anti-inflammatory. Since it is relatively cheap, and has been around forever, it is seldom actively marketed. Yet, since its introduction as a therapeutic agent in 1957, hundreds of scientific papers have appeared in medical literature attesting to its effectiveness. Bromelain has proven effective in treating allergies, arthritis, bronchitis, cellulitis, contusions, degenerative joint diseases, pancreatic insufficiency, sinusitis, sprains, strains, tumors and more (Taussig S. and Batkin S.; Bromelain, the Enzyme Complex of Pineapple and Its Clinical Application; Journal of Ethnopharmacol 22, 1988).

One study compared bromelain against NSAID's for treatment of osteoarthritis of the knee. While both groups received equal benefit in pain reduction and improved mobility, the bromelain was the substance without potentially dangerous side effects, showing it to be a viable alternative to the pharmaceutical approach (Klein G. and Kullich W.; Short-Term Treatment of Painful Osteoarthritis of the Knee With Oral Enzymes; W Clinical Drug Investigation; Jan 2000).

Bromelain reduces inflammation via a process called "fibrinolysis." In this process, bromelain stimulates the production of plasmin, which breaks down fibrin deposits, and prevents fibrin from producing swelling, as the plasmin blocks the formation of inflammatory compounds. Varicose veins have built-up fibrin deposits in the tissue near the veins, causing the skin surrounding the vein to become lumpy and hard. Inability of the body to break down fibrin is linked to an increased risk of mycocardial infarction, pulmonary embolism, thrombophlebitis (vein inflammation) and stroke.

SERRATIA PEPTIDASE

The Serratia protease (or proteolytic enzyme) is marketed under many different, similar sounding names, and is well researched in Japan and Europe. It seems to have a broader ability than bromelain in the digesting of non-living tissue (arterial plaque, blood clots, cysts and fibrin). Most of the actual studies done on this enzyme, however, are based on treating inflammation and pain due to physical trauma, especially post-operative trauma (Esch PM., Gerngross H. and Fabian A.; Reduction of Postoperative Swelling; Fortschr Med. 1989).

Other clinical studies showed effectiveness in treating breast engorgement, respiratory ailments and sinusitis. In fact, though this enzyme is often marketed for arthritic conditions, most of the research quoted to support the sales of serratia peptidase products, was done with bromelain (by Dr. Hans Nieper). Though, a recent study from India did confirm its effectiveness on carpal tunnel syndrome, showing significant clinical improvement in 65% of the case subjects (Dept. of Neurology, SMS Medical College and Hospital; A Preliminary Trial of Serratiopeptidase in Patients With Carpal Tunnel Syndrome; J Assoc Physicians India; Nov 2000).

ENTERIC COATING?

The necessity of enteric coating (covering the pill with a substance that resists stomach acid) proteolytic enzymes, when they are to be used to reduce inflammation, or remove cellular debris from the body, is debatable. Aside from the marketing hype, a scientific perspective indicates that enteric-coating is not actually necessary. Indeed, some studies have indicated that non-enteric coated protease products are more effective than enteric-coated ones (see above: "Bromelain, the Enzyme Complex of Pineapple and Its Clinical Application"; Bromelain is seldom enteric-coated in clinical studies).

Since the first function of protein digesting enzymes is to digest protein, if these enzymes are ingested while there is protein in the stomach that is what they will do. If there is no protein in the stomach, they will move on to their secondary functions of reducing inflammation and cleaning out waste materials. So, when using non-enteric-coated protease products, simply take them away from protein: ingest either on an empty stomach (half an hour before eating, or one hour after eating), or with fruit or carbohydrates, but no protein (meat, fish, eggs, poultry, dairy, tofu, tempeh, etc).

CONTRAINDICATIONS

Bromelain and serratia peptidase will increase the concentration of antibiotics in the bloodstream. While, in an ideal system, this could allow for less antibiotics to be used (if they were properly prescribed together), it can be dangerous to mix the two without professional medical advice. Bromelain reduces blood platelet aggregation and so should not be combined with blood thinning medications, without the guidance of a medical professional. All protein digesting enzymes can irritate existing ulcers, and so should be avoided by those with either intestinal or stomach ulcers.

ANTI-INFLAMMATORY HERBS

Many different herbs, from different areas of the world, have anti-inflammatory properties, and have been used for centuries for such purposes. These include Alfalfa, Boswellia, Devil's Claw, Ginger, Green Tea, Turmeric and Yucca. We have devoted a chapter to Green Tea, but here's a quick look at the others.

ALFALFA

Alfalfa both detoxifies and alkalizes the body. It is used in folk medicine to treat arthritic and rheumatoid conditions, including lower back pain and sciatica. In Chinese medicine, Alfalfa is a "cooling" tonic, useful for treating acute and chronic inflammatory symptoms associated with degeneration and aging. Alfalfa contains saponins, which cleans out the joints, allowing room for new cartilage growth. Often the joints have become occupied with cellular debris (uric acid crystals and calcium deposits). This build-up is the reason many people often do not find relief from glucosamine, and other cartilage rebuilding supplements. Saponins are detergent-like compounds that gradually clean out the joints, allowing room for the rebuilding agents to get in and do their job. Bromelain has also shown the ability to break down uric acid crystals.

BOSWELLIA

Boswellia (Boswellia carterii) resin is derived from the frankincense tree, found growing in India, and has a long history of use in the Middle East. It is a natural COX-2 inhibitor and has shown good results in treating osteoarthritis, rheumatoid arthritis and ulcerative colitis. It will shrink inflamed tissue, increase blood supply to inflamed joints, and repair blood vessels damaged by inflammation. It also appears to stimulate some cartilage growth, as well.

DEVIL'S CLAW

The extract of Devil's Claw (Harpagophytum procumbens) is most commonly used to treat rheumatoid arthritis, but is has very broad anti-inflammatory properties, and can also reduce pain levels. Studies indicate that this South African herb can be effectively used to treat arthritis, carpal tunnel syndrome, gout and tendonitis. The majority of testing on Devil's Claw has been done on treating lower back pain, where it has shown to be most effective on severe cases. Like many of the herbs that relieve pain and inflammation, Devil's Claw contains compounds that improve circulation and remove inflammatory chemicals from damaged tissues. It can relax the arteries, in effect reducing blood pressure, but since it can also reduce the force of the heartbeat and pulse, Devil's Claw is to be used only with advice from a professional if you have congestive heart failure.

GINGER

Ginger has been used for over 2000 years as a remedy for inflammation and pain, since it curbs the chemicals in the body that create a long-term tendency toward inflammation. Ginger is a natural COX-2 inhibitor with strong antioxidant properties, and is the perfect food to use on a daily basis, as seasoning or tea, to keep inflammation in check. In a clinical study with arthritis patients, 75 % of the participants using ginger, reported substantial improvement including pain relief, increased joint mobility, and decreased swelling and morning stiffness. Ginger's ability to inhibit the formation of inflammatory prostaglandins is complemented by its function of improving circulation.

TURMERIC

Turmeric (curcuma longa), a powerful source of antioxidants, is well proven to reduce inflammation, help prevent some cancers and to protect the liver. To Ayurvedic (East Indian) medicine, Turmeric, aside from its use as a spice, was considered to be a cleansing herb for detoxifying the whole body. In traditional Chinese medicine it is used for liver and gallbladder ailments, to stop bleeding, reduce lung congestion and treat menstrual problems.

In clinical studies, extracts from Turmeric have shown an effectiveness in reducing inflammation that is comparable to corticosteroids, but without side effects. Inflammatory conditions successfully treated with Turmeric, and extracts from it, include arthritis, bursitis, carpel tunnel syndrome, eczema, endometriosis and tendonitis. The enzyme Bromelain has a synergistic effect when combined with Turmeric, dramatically enhancing its absorption in the body.

Because Turmeric requires large amounts to be effective (a tbsp per day), most products use the 95% standardized "Curcumin" extract. It has been found, however, that isolated Curcumin can actually increase free radical production, when it is not balanced by the other components found in the whole plant. If you are going to use a Turmeric product for a long time, it should be standardized to 95% "Curcuminoids," which contains concentrated aspects of the whole Turmeric plant, giving us the full range of benefits, with no possible side effects.

Turmeric compounds have also been shown to reduce heart disease and cancer. For the heart, Turmeric reduces atherosclerosis, preventing cholesterol from building up into arterial plaque, relaxes blood vessels lowering the risk of stroke, and protects the heart from tissue damage, if a heart attack does occur. In laboratory cancer studies, Curcumin will kill leukemia cells and reduce the spread of tumors. It has specific benefit for preventing and treating oral cancer, colorectal cancer and melanoma, and reduces lung cancer rates in tobacco smokers. Turmeric and its extracts also have a good track record in preventing and treating cataracts, gallstones, bad breath, gum disease and indigestion.

YUCCA

This herb (Yucca schidigera) has been used by Southwestern Native Americans for centuries as a treatment for pain and inflammation, due to arthritic conditions. Yucca is also used to enhance immune function and to treat allergies. In a study with arthritic patients, at least 60% of the participants reported diminished pain, stiffness and swelling, without any side effects (Dr. Robert Bingham, Journal of Applied Nutrition, Vol 27, No. 2 & 3).

Yucca includes properties that decrease bacteria endotoxin absorption, which can improve cartilage synthesis. In double blind studies, it has been shown to be effective in the management of arthritis. It has been suggested that these effects are due to protecting and improving levels of gastrointestinal flora ("friendly bacteria"). Bacterial endotoxins (toxic byproducts or harmful bacteria) have been shown to depress the biosynthesis of cartilage and to create allergic responses. We see that this mechanism is the same one referred to at the beginning of this chapter, with regards to soluble fiber, and how it can lower C-reactive protein levels.

Yucca is also rich in saponins, which as we saw with Alfalfa, help to clean out waste deposits from the joints. Saponins also aid in digestion and the absorption of fats, so when saponins were given in an extract form to patients for 6 months or longer, all showed a normalizing of blood cholesterol and triglyceride levels, along with improved blood pressure levels (Dr. Robert Bingham, Arthritis News Today, Vol 2, No 6).

CHAPTER SEVEN

PROTECTING THE PROSTATE

JUST FOR MEN?

Excited by a new weapon in our arsenal against rampant prostate disorders, this chapter will touch on the basics of current prostate treatment, and then introduce this new agent.

This one may appear to be for men only but, aside from reading it for the man in your life, there is another reason that women may wish to read this chapter. That is because, for menopausal women, the mechanism that causes hair loss is much the same as that which causes prostate swelling, and hair loss, in men.

This mechanism is based on excessive testosterone, and its tendency to breakdown into damaging byproducts: the process commonly known as "male-pattern baldness." When a woman is in menopause, her reduced estrogen level has the effect of essentially raising the relative amount of testosterone that is circulating in her body. Therefore women experiencing hair loss, as a side effect of menopause, may safely try the herbal remedies that are recommended to shrink the male prostate gland (of these, my best feedback has been with "beta-sitosterol"). As well, some of the ancillary benefits of the aforementioned "new weapon" have applications for both genders (cholesterol and blood pressure problems), and anecdotal evidence suggesting it to be effective at treating symptoms of menopause and incontinence in women.

First let's get a look at that prostate. The prostate is a cluster of small, doughnut-shaped sex glands. They encircle the urethra (the tube which conveys urine and semen) just below the bladder. Though all the functions of the prostate are not yet clear, its most direct purpose is to contract during ejaculation, squeezing the seminal fluid into and through the urethral tract. Because the prostate encircles the urethra, any problem with the prostate can hinder the free flow of urine.

BPH and DHT

Approximately 50% of men between the ages of 40 and 60 have the most common disorder of the prostate gland; benign prostatic hyperplasia (BPH). Symptoms of BPH include increased frequency of urination, waking at night to empty the bladder, and reduced force and caliber of urination. It is believed that BPH is caused by an accumulation of testosterone in the prostate. Within the prostate, the enzyme known as 5-alpha reductase converts the male sex hormone, testosterone, into another more potent hormone, known as dihydrotestosterone (DHT), the same hormone linked to causing Male Pattern Baldness.

DHT controls the division of cells in the prostate, and when there is too much DHT it stimulates the prostate cells to multiply excessively, eventually causing the prostate to enlarge. Normally, DHT would be excreted from the prostate gland in sufficient quantity to prevent enlargement. If, however, there is an imbalance between the male hormones (androgens), then the DHT is not adequately excreted, causing the prostate to swell. Examination of an enlarged prostate usually reveals the presence of three to four times the normal levels of DHT.

PROSTATITIS

The second most common ailment of the prostate is prostatitis, which is a swelling of the prostate, caused by bacterial infection.

This can occur at any age, and the symptoms are more severe than those of BPH. It begins with irritation during urination, then pain between the scrotum and rectum, pain in the lower back and ultimately, blood in the urine. Urine flow can be partially or totally blocked, which can lead to urine retention in the bladder, in turn causing urinary infections. Protracted urine retention can also cause damage to the "ureters" (the ducts that carry the urine from a kidney to the bladder), as the urine backs up into the kidneys.

It now appears that a new cause of chronic prostatitis is the accumulation of nickel in the prostate gland. Nickel is a trace element that is becoming a heavy metal due to being excessively available in the environment. Apparently bacteria thrive on nickel.

Nickel is found in tobacco smoke, vegetable shortenings (especially deep-fryer fat) and pesticide residue, but it is likely that its current increase in the body is due to cheap, Chinese stainless steel cookware. Stainless steel comes in many different grades, and the cheaper grades are made from many different alloys. These include nickel and chromium, which are now believed to bleed into foods, when they react with the salts and acids of the foods cooked in them. In order to avoid most of this, do not allow acidic or salty foods to remain in the steel cookware for long periods of time.

True stainless steel cookware should be of the highest-grade surgical steel, which is known as 316L, and is the grade mandated for use by the dairy and pharmaceutical industries. 304 is another designation for high end steel to look for. The old terminology for surgical stainless steel was 18/10, meaning that the chromium level is between 16 and 18%, and the nickel content is between 10 and 15%. This designation is still often used on cookware and indicates a superior grade of steel.

As a result of this new finding, treatment for chronic prostatitis has now incorporated the amino acid "L-histidine" (at 500 to 1500mg daily). This amino acid seems to bind to nickel and chelate (pull) it out of the body through the urine, though it can take many months before this is accomplished. Histidine has a long track record of use as a chelating agent for copper, iron and other heavy metals. Dosages have ranged between 1 and 6 grams daily. It has been used to treat arthritis, allergies, nerve deafness, and has been found to be necessary for the maintenance of the myelin sheaths (which protect nerve endings).

A non-bacterial form of prostatitis also can also occur. Some researchers believe that this form of prostatitis is caused by a build-up of uric acid crystals, the same process that causes gout. (See previous chapter for info on removing uric acid deposits.)

For prostatitis where infection is involved, the eating of blueberries or cranberries (or concentrated capsules of them) can prevent e-coli bacteria from attaching to the lining of the prostate. During infection one should not take iron supplements (and avoid red meat which is both high in iron and contributes to uric acid build-up), as iron feeds bacteria in the body. This holds true for all forms of infection in the body. Also avoid items that are irritating to the bladder, including alcohol, coffee, citrus juices and spicy foods.

The greatest danger that follows either BPH or prostatitis problems, is that of a possible malignant change occurring. The metabolites (breakdown products) of cholesterol are cancer producing and have a tendency to accumulate in the prostate gland. These metabolites initiate degeneration in the prostate cells, which can promote prostatic enlargement and sometimes cancer.

PROSTATE CANCER

It is interesting to note that as little as a hundred years ago, prostate problems were rarely mentioned in medical literature. This implies a link to the modern lifestyle: most likely to diet. Indeed, the connection between diet and prostate cancer has been clearly established; there is a high correlation between prostate cancer and fat consumption.

Worldwide autopsies reveal that wherever the diet is similar to a typical North American one (i.e. high in animal fat consumption) nearly 25% of all men develop latent cancer of the prostate by the time they reach their senior years. American research includes the "NIH-AARP Diet and Health Study," which tracked 175,000 men (age 50 and up) over nine years. Researchers from the U.S. National Cancer Institute concluded that prostate cancer risk was approximately 30% higher among those who ate the most red meat (130 grams daily) versus those who ate the least (25 grams daily). Risk factor also went up about 30% in the men who consumed the most processed meat (containing nitrites, a preservative), and among those who consumed the most barbequed or grilled meats (which contain benzopyrene, a carcinogen resulting from browning or blackening proteins).

A few years ago, The Journal of the National Cancer Institute reported that men who ate red meat at least five times a week, had a two and a half times greater risk of developing prostate cancer, than did men who ate red meat less than once a week (based on a study of 51,000 men). A study by the Chief of Urology at the Metropolitan Hospital in New York, found that men with BPH had 80% more cholesterol in their blood, than those without the condition. Remember that sex hormones, including testosterone, are built in the body from cholesterol.

Maintaining safe cholesterol levels obviously involves watching saturated fat consumption, but it also must include restricting sugar intake and ensuring an adequate amount of fiber. Both sugar and fiber are involved in the body's ability to process and utilize cholesterol. Another good reason to include high fiber content in your diet is the need for bowel regularity.

Constipation is a frequent symptom accompanying BPH. It is implied that the long-term increase in pressure from constipation, creates congestion in the lower pelvic region, where the prostate lies. Putrefying matter in this area can also contribute to prostatitis, as constipation produces a cesspool of bad bacteria, which can infect the prostate gland. Thus it is important to take a good quality probiotic (acidophilus) on a regular basis, if we have any irregularity problems.

One of the best dietary choices to prevent prostate cancer is the consumption of cruciferous vegetables. Many studies over the last few decades have confirmed a general anti-cancer effect from these vegetables, which include broccoli, cauliflower and cabbage. Now, lab studies have shown a particular protective effect of certain cruciferous compounds on prostate cancer. A lecture given at the American Association for Cancer Research, by Dr. Shivendra Singh, showed these phytonutrients ("isothiocyanates") to reduce cancer growth in prostate tumors and to inhibit angiogenisis (the new blood vessels that grow and spread tumors) in prostate cancer cells.

PSA TESTING

It must be mentioned that, 20 years ago the approach to prostate cancer was, "you'll die of old age before prostate cancer kills you." At some point in the last few decades the medical profession started diagnosing and treating prostate cancer, and it is now one of the leading causes of death among men. The primary tool used to track the health of the prostate, aside from the finger test (digital rectal exam) that the doctor uses to check for BPH, is the PSA (prostate-specific antigen) test.

The validity of this test has been questioned for some time now, but even more so with the release of two large international studies in March '09. Following the release of these studies the Canadian Cancer Society announced: "Not only does it not appear to reduce death rates from prostate cancer overall, but there are significant harms associated with prostate cancer testing with PSA." The "harms" mentioned refer to the unnecessary surgery that may then occur, leading to many men suffering with incontinence and impotence, following treatment. Such routine screening for prostate cancer ultimately lead to over one million men in the United States being treated for "tumors growing too slowly to do any harm" (Vancouver Sun; Feb 3, 2010).

While this prostate produced protein may indicate prostate cancer, when found at high levels in the blood, it may also indicate infection, irritation or BPH, and, one may have prostate cancer without having elevated PSA levels. A further debatable action is the biopsy following the high PSA reading. This invasive technique punches holes in the prostate to accumulate enough matter to biopsy, meanwhile causing pain, bleeding and inflammation. As cancer is in part an inflammatory condition, subjecting a delicate organ to this abuse could even cause a worsening and/or spreading of what cancerous cells may be present.

DANGERS OF THE PSA TEST

In the two studies that questioned the effectiveness of PSA testing, men aged 55 and older were followed for approximately a decade (75,000 in the American study and 182,000 in the European study), in both cases half the men received PSA tests and half did not. The prostate cancer death rate "was very low and did not differ significantly" between the two groups of men, and the PSA test "was associated with a high risk of over-diagnosis." "All and all it is really not a very effective tool to screen for prostate cancer," said Heather Logan, a senior director at the Canadian Cancer Society.

And new data suggests, that the diagnosis of prostate cancer alone dramatically increases the risk of suicide and death from heart attack. Published in the Journal of the National Cancer Institute, was a large study done on 340,000 men who had been diagnosed with prostate cancer, between the years 1979 and 2004. The study, done at Harvard and Brigham & Women's Hospital in Boston, examined the first year following the diagnosis, and saw a 90% increase in suicide risk, and a doubling of risk for heart attacks and strokes. This was no surprise, as it has already been found that stress from any sudden calamity (such as an earthquake) can increase heart attack rates.

While this study claimed that the elevated risk of suicide occurred mostly before the advent of standard PSA testing, in roughly 1993, it still saw "an increased risk for cardiovascular death, which is about 60 % greater in that first month after diagnosis." And, a Swedish study recently found PSA testing still associated with increased suicide risk. The conclusion of such studies is that the high stress associated with the diagnosis of prostate cancer, needs to be countered by counseling and support afterwards.

Evidently, the PSA test has its place as one form of feedback, to be balanced out by other diagnostic techniques, but should not be relied upon singly, as being the determinant of prostate cancer. A proficient doctor will use it as a guide, observing it over years and, if the levels are constantly rising over time, other tests may be called for, before we get to the biopsy and treatment phase.

SUPPLEMENTS FOR THE PROSTATE

MINERALS

So, what is the natural approach to support our little buddy, the prostate gland? Let's start with the most important nutrient needed by men and their prostate gland, which is zinc. Men have twice the zinc needs of women, as women have twice the iron needs of men (as explained in Part One: Gender Differences; see also Chapter Six under "Minerals" for more information on zinc).

Zinc has been shown to inhibit the activity of "5-alpha reductase," the enzyme that converts testosterone to DHT, leading to BPH. Levels of zinc are commonly inadequate in the average male, leading to higher 5-alpha reductase levels. The prostate gland normally contains about ten times more zinc than any other organ in the body. As a preventative supplement 15mg to 30mg per day is usually sufficient.

The older you are the more zinc you need, and if you have a prostate infection you may require levels up to 50mg per day, to help fight the infection. Levels of 30mg or more daily should be taken with a small amount of copper (one or two milligrams), if used on an ongoing basis, since high zinc intake can deplete the body of copper, as a high intake of copper will deplete zinc. (I have even seen this occur in a woman, whose zinc deficiency was apparently caused by her copper I.U.D.) Vitamin B-6 is also required for the absorption of zinc.

One of the most important nutrients to prevent prostate cancer is the mineral selenium. Researchers found cadmium (a heavy metal) concentrations in the prostate of those with BPH, to be considerably higher than in normal tissue, with the DHT level directly proportional to cadmium concentrations. Although other investigators failed to confirm these findings, prostatic hyperplasia has been produced in animals by injecting cadmium into the prostate. As well, in laboratory experiments, cadmium stimulates the overgrowth of human prostatic epithelium (a sign of cancer). In these studies, the correct concentration of selenium inhibited cadmium-stimulated prostatic growth. As selenium intake is frequently inadequate in the Western diet, supplementing with 100mcg to 200mcg daily is a good idea.

Boron is a trace mineral, commonly used to maintain bone mass, when taken along with calcium, and has had some success in treating arthritis. It appears that boron is required for the conversion of vitamin D to its active form in the body, which would be the link between boron and osteoporosis and arthritis. As I covered in Part One, vitamin D deficiency has been rampant in North America, up until just recently. In that chapter, it was also noted that vitamin D deficiency is clearly linked to prostate cancer. If boron deficiency is added to vitamin D deficiency, we can see how it would compound these conditions. For the prostate, boron has shown some promise as an anti-cancer agent. We know that it helps to regulate estrogen and testosterone in women, so it may be of hormonal help to men as well, but at the very least, it will help to maintain healthy PSA levels. A usual dose is between 1.5mg and 3mg per day.

HERBS AND PLANT STEROLS

Nettle root extract has been used successfully to exert a decongestive action on the prostate, thus relieving the discomfort caused by the enlargement of this gland. The vitamins, minerals and lipids found in Nettles have been shown to inhibit the activity of 5-alpha reductase, as well as supporting endocrine gland activity. Nettle root also protects the prostate from excess estrogen, which becomes more common as men age. It is only the root of this plant that benefits the prostate, so avoid prostate products that use the leaf, since it indicates that they haven't done their research. The leaves however do have value elsewhere, including treating allergies.

But, the first choice in treating BPH is the use of a standardized, fat-soluble extract of the fruit of the Saw Palmetto plant. This extract is effective at preventing the conversion of testosterone to DHT, and also inhibits the binding of DHT to cellular receptor sites, thereby increasing the breakdown and excretion of DHT. Saw Palmetto has solid research supporting its ability to shrink swollen prostate tissue, including studies done in Britain, Italy and Germany. For women, it has historical use for enlarging the breasts, and as a treatment for menopausal induced hirsutism (unwanted body hair). It is suggested, however, that women taking hormone-regulating drugs (birth control pills and HRT) should avoid saw palmetto, due to possible interactions. This also holds true for men on prescription prostate drugs. A therapeutic dose of Saw Palmetto is 160mg of a standardized extract taken twice per day: a maintenance dose being about half as much.

Next to Saw Palmetto, the herb most renown for protecting the prostate is Pygeum. In a European double-blind study that involved almost 700 men, Pygeum worked to alleviate symptoms in 66% of the cases. Native to Africa, Pygeum (prunus africanum) reduces blood concentrations of luteinizing hormone and testosterone, forbidding the swollen prostate gland from absorbing them and thereby worsening the condition. It also reduces inflammatory agents and the hormone prolactin (linked to prostate problems), and blocks cholesterol from the prostate. Bad news for men; beer raises prolactin, which is linked to depression as well as prostate swelling. This is because the hops in the beer are estrogenic (prolactin is considered a "female" hormone), and the older men get the worse it is for them, since andropause (the male version of menopause) is caused by a decline in male hormones, along with an elevation of female hormones.

While Pygeum is often included in Saw Palmetto formulas, it should be noted that Pygeum can be effective for treating prostate infection, whereas Saw Palmetto is not. Therefore, if prostatitis is the concern, one should focus on getting a higher dose of Pygeum than Saw Palmetto. Dosage is approximately about 50mg to 100mg of a standardized extract, twice per day. Both BPH and non-bacterial prostatitis have been shown to respond well to a specific, mechanically harvested pollen extract (sold under different trade names, including "Cernitin"). This follows on the heels of the traditional use of general bee pollen (one to two teaspoons daily) to support prostate health, treat prostate conditions, and balance male hormones. (In the area of "bee-foods," Royal Jelly tends to work better for balancing female hormones.)

Phytosterols are cholesterol analogs found in vegetables, which decrease cholesterol absorption by displacing cholesterol from bile salt. At one point about 50 years ago, phytosterols were used as a drug for lowering cholesterol, and did so safely and effectively. An extract of one phytosterol, Beta-Sitosterol, has been studied for the treatment of BPH, under double-blind conditions, and in most studies has shown efficacy. Dosage levels are from 200mg to 300mg daily. A further advantage to Beta-Sitosterol is that in laboratory experiments, it was able to reduce prostate cancer cell growth by 24% and quadruple cancerous cell death.

AMINO ACIDS

Studies have found a specific combination of amino acids (L-glutamic acid 530 mg, L-alanine 200 mg and glycine 90 mg), taken 3 times daily, to have some therapeutic value. More than 90% of subjects in these studies experienced reduction in residual urine and shrinkage of the prostate. The effectiveness of this combination has become so well accepted, that has been used as the "control drug" against which to test other, possibly therapeutic, substances for the prostate.

Glycine alone also has a good track record for treating BPH. I had a client who was a gentleman in his fifties, and I started him on a natural growth hormone enhancing product, in order to increase his energy levels and to reduce some body fat. This product was based on 6 grams of L-glycine (the level at which it has been shown to elevate growth hormone levels). While it takes a month or more to notice the increased growth hormone levels, he returned within two weeks to tell me a positive side-effect that had occurred; he stopped having to get up at night to urinate. He had already tried zinc and saw palmetto-based products, to no avail, and so was thrilled to report that, for some reason, this product had done the trick.

Glycine, a non-essential amino acid, is found in considerable amounts in prostate fluid. Studies on glycine and BPH have found benefit at doses as low as 800mg daily, but it now appears that it should be avoided by those with prostate cancer. In 2009 researchers reported that the amino acid "sarcosine" when found in high levels in the body, corresponded with increased progression of prostate cancer. Sarcosine is built in the body through the combination of glycine and methionine (found mostly in red meat), so it has been suggested that those with prostate cancer should avoid glycine. As well, it was found that deficiency in vitamin B2 (riboflavin) and folic acid also lead to the buildup of high sarcosine levels.

MULTI-CAROTENOIDS

And now to the exciting "new weapon" in our arsenal against prostate disorders. Recently, a new botanical drug was listed in the USA 2009 Physicians' Desk Reference. Known as "L-O-M Multi-Carotenoids," this unique mixture of carotenoids, including Lycopene, has been used for over ten years in Asia and Europe, for treating BHP, high cholesterol, hypertension and female urinary incontinence. Shown to be more effective than saw palmetto for BPH, these multi-carotenoids have also been proven to be more effective than Lycopene at protecting the prostate against cancer.

Even though lycopene is commonly used as a supplement to protect the prostate gland from cancer, the American FDA has determined that lycopene, in isolation, does not have the benefits that it does when in its natural state (in stewed tomatoes, for example). When approached to allow health claims regarding lycopene, and risk reduction for some forms of cancer, the FDA concluded: "there was no credible evidence to support an association between lycopene intake and a reduced risk of prostate and other cancers." They found that intake of cooked tomatoes (ideally with some fat in it) was inversely associated with prostate cancer risk, but found no relationship between intake of raw tomatoes and prostate cancer risk. Unlike isolated or synthesized lycopene, the L-O-M Multi-Carotenoids contain a naturally extracted family of carotenoids, complex in structure, like whole foods. This is why it can do what lycopene alone cannot.

In an American clinical trial on prostate cancer patients, after three weeks of supplementing with L-O-M Multi-Carotenoids

(30mg/day), before prostatectomy, PSA levels in the supplementation group decreased by 18%, while in the placebo group they increased by 14%. There is only one other natural substance, to my knowledge, that can lower PSA levels, and this is an uncommon, very specific extract of rye pollen (Cernitin).

When we look back to the beginning of this article, we can see another benefit of the L-O-M product for helping to further protect the prostate against cancer, and that is with regards to lowering cholesterol. An animal study done in 2007 concluded that L-O-M caused an increase of 28.6% in HDL ("good" cholesterol) levels, and dramatically reduced total cholesterol, triglycerides and LDL ("bad" cholesterol) levels. The icing on the cake is the powerful antioxidant effect that these multi-carotenoids have, effectively raising blood levels of SOD (Superoxide Dismutase), CAT (Catalase) and GSH (Glutathione Stimulating Hormone).

Since these internally-produced antioxidants protect us against all forms of cancer, heart disease, premature aging and many diseases, the benefits of L-O-M multi-Carotenoids extend well beyond the prostate gland, and beyond the gender of male. More specifically for women, feedback from gynecologists and naturopaths showed a prompt, positive response from women experiencing urinary incontinence, or frequent urination due to prolapsed bladder and uterus. It has also shown success in treating menopausal symptoms, as this testimonial from Canada indicates: "...With L-O-M the hot flushes and night sweats are gone. The insomnia and mood swings have abated significantly to a tolerable level."

In Canada L-O-M is available through Naturopaths, or found in vitamin stores under the name PROSTChoice. It is designed to be taken on an on-going basis for both preventive care (12mg daily) or for treatment (15mg to 30mg).

CONCLUSION

In closing, I would like to comment on a recent newspaper editorial (The Vancouver Sun; Feb 6, 2010), that serves as a reminder not to take our freedom to supplement for granted. This editorial opens with something I have already discussed, namely that "you can get too much of a good thing, and vitamins are no exception." Referencing a study published in "Annals of Pharmacotherapy," co-authored by a pediatric emergency specialist (Ran Goldman), the editors warn us that some vitamins can be dangerous. The study was designed to assess adverse effects associated with the use of vitamins, and the possible interactions of vitamins with drugs. It suggests that certain nutrients can be problematic if children are given higher than the "recommended doses" by parents, who then don't inform their pediatric physicians that the children are taking these vitamins. Specifically mentioned are vitamins A, D, E, folic acid and niacin.

The author's solution to this potentially dangerous dosing of children, supported by the editorial, is that these vitamins be categorized as over the counter medications. This would make parents take the issue more seriously and would mandate that these vitamins be labeled with recommended doses, and warnings about interactions with other medications.

On the surface, this appears to be a reasonable approach, since who can argue with protecting our children? Let's overlook the fact that the current Canadian regulatory body, the NHPD (Natural Health Products Directorate), is in the process of having all supplements labeled in such a manner, including recommended doses for appropriate ages, all possible interactions with medications, and any allergenic potential. In fact, the main reason for this new agency, designed to regulate the supplement industry, was to create a class separate from drugs; acknowledging that vitamins and supplements are somewhere between food and drug, and should be treated as such. With more caution than food and less than with drugs.

If we were to backslide to the point where we allowed basic nutritional supplements to be categorized as medications, then it is a short slippery slope to allowing them to be restricted to prescription only. Before the NHPD existed, all vitamins and minerals (but not herbs) had to have a D.I.N. (drug identification number), which was tantamount to admitting that they were drug-like. This approach has now been changed in Canada, due to consistent work by many concerned citizens, non-profit groups and industry representatives. These groups, finally, got the government to create a new regulatory body to patrol the industry, without destroying it. The battle, however, is not yet won, as initially the NHPD was holding supplements to pharmaceutical standards and requiring clinical studies that were similar to drug studies, in order for approval to be sold. Currently the system is back on track and most supplements in Canada have a fair chance at receiving a license, with the advantage of now being able to make claims on the label (something previously forbidden).

Let's have a quick look the danger these hypothetical children were put into. Vitamin A, at high doses has been linked to "abdominal discomfort" and "liver damage"; too much vitamin D can cause "headaches, fatigue, weakness" and "anemia and kidney stones"; large doses of vitamin E or niacin could "increase the chances of bleeding in children taking ibuprofen"; excessive folic acid and niacin can "reduce the effectiveness of epilepsy medications."

Now, how many parents do you think would give adult doses of supplements to children? And, since most adults cannot even manage high doses of niacin, because of the intense flush, how and why, would you give it to children? If your child was on an epilepsy medication, do you not think that you would have the common sense to tell your physician if you were giving them anything more than a children's one-a-day?

The potential dangers here are both dubious and unlikely to occur, except in the most rare of conditions. Warnings on the label: by all means. But, calling a vitamin a medication is like calling a man with a library fine a dangerous offender. Let's put the dangers into proper perspective and label them as such. Pharmaceutical drugs are dangerous. Period. Supplements should be used with caution, but are not dangerous. Except calcium, which is only so because we listened to medical advice on how to use it. So, the conclusion is, never take a doctor's advice on supplements. If you need advice on pharmaceuticals, talk to a pharmacist, who will give you better advice than a doctor, since that is his area of expertise, and he has an overview that is not based on the latest drug marketing material, that physicians are constantly bombarded with.

Finally, remember the words usually attributed to Thomas Jefferson (though this is debatable): "The price of freedom is eternal vigilance." Keep pressure on your government representatives so they know that voters are paying attention. Anyone can send a message, no postage required, to their Member of Parliament, by name, to House of Commons, Ottawa, Ontario, K1A 0A6. Remind them of your right to make informed personal decisions and choices affecting your health, and that you wish to continue to have access to Natural Health Products currently available without prescription or restriction.

This concludes our first tour of modern health data. In the

books to follow, I plan on moving into more unusual and obscure information, no less valuable but somewhat more advanced, than what is contained in this book. Each of the other two projected books will be designed to build upon this one, just as we build a basic nutritional foundation, before we move on to the treatments more specific to our individual health concerns. And, as we strive for optimal health and longevity, it is important to remember that obsessing over it is counter-productive. Many people forget that the saying "moderation in all things" ends with, "including moderation." As some wise man once said, "it is better to eat pizza with friends, than brown rice alone."